An Atlas of Imaging of the Paranasal Sinuses

In Memory of

Padmanabhan Rangaswamy

1923–1992

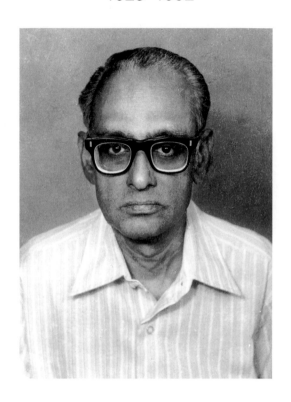

An Atlas of Imaging of the Paranasal Sinuses

Lalitha Shankar

Department of Diagnostic Imaging
University of Toronto
St Joseph's Health Centre
Toronto
Canada

Kathryn Evans

Ear, Nose and Throat Department
St Bartholomew's Hospital
London
United Kingdom

Michael Hawke

Department of Otorhinolaryngology
University of Toronto
Canada

Heinz Stammberger

University Ear, Nose and Throat Hospital
Graz
Austria

MARTIN DUNITZ

Color photographs © Lalitha Shankar, Kathryn
Evans, Michael Hawke, Heinz Stammberger 1994

First published in the United Kingdom in 1994
by Martin Dunitz Ltd, The Livery House,
7–9 Pratt Street, London NW1 0AE

A CIP catalogue record for this book is available
from the British Library.

ISBN 1 85317 124 7

Originated by Scribe Design, Gillingham, Kent
Color origination by Imago Publishing Ltd
Manufactured by Imago Publishing Ltd
Printed and bound in Singapore

Contents

Contributors

Kathryn Evans

Ear, Nose and Throat Department, St Bartholomew's Hospital, London, United Kingdom

Michael Hawke

Department of Otorhinolaryngology, University of Toronto, Canada

David Kirkpatrick

Department of Otolaryngology, Dalhousie University, Halifax, Canada

Ludger Klimek

Department of Otorhinolaryngology, Plastic Surgery of the Head and Neck, Medical Faculty, Aachen Technical University, Germany

Neal Lofchy

Department of Otorhinolaryngology, University of Toronto, Canada

Martyn Mendelsohn

Department of Otorhinolaryngology, Mount Sinai Hospital, University of Toronto, Canada

Ralph Mösges

Department of Otorhinolaryngology, Plastic Surgery of the Head and Neck, Medical Faculty, Aachen Technical University, Germany

Arnold Noyek

Department of Otorhinolaryngology and Department of Radiology, University of Toronto; Department of Otorhinolaryngology, Mount Sinai Hospital, Toronto, Canada

Michael Riding

Department of Radiology, Dalhousie University, Halifax, Canada

Lalitha Shankar

Department of Diagnostic Imaging, University of Toronto, St Joseph's Health Centre, Toronto, Canada

Heinz Stammberger

University Ear, Nose and Throat Hospital, Graz, Austria

John Stevens

The Eye Institute, Toronto Western Division, The Toronto Hospital, Canada

Judy Trogadis

Volume Investigation Laboratory, Toronto Western Division, The Toronto Hospital, University of Toronto, Canada

Sunil Ummat

Department of Otolaryngology, Dalhousie University, Halifax, Canada

Preface

This atlas attempts to provide a comprehensive review of the current imaging modalities that play an important role in the management of sinonasal disease. Computed tomography (CT) and magnetic resonance (MR) imaging have revolutionized the diagnosis of diseases of the paranasal sinuses. These imaging techniques can generate images in any desired plane. This atlas will familiarize the reader with the normal anatomy and the common pathological entities as seen by these modalities. It will also enable the otorhinolaryngologist to become competent in interpretation of CT and/or MR images. We hope that practicing radiologists who wish to develop greater proficiency in the interpretation of the various anatomic variants, pathology and postoperative changes in the paranasal sinuses will use this book to enhance their clinical knowledge.

It is obvious that technology continuously plays a leading role in the practice of medicine. New techniques constantly change the management of various disorders: CT and MR images are the present-day gold standards in the management of paranasal sinus disease.

LS
MH
KE
HS

Acknowledgments

This book would not have been possible without the co-operation and the enthusiasm of several individuals. We include their names as a small token of appreciation for all their efforts in making it possible.

We wish to thank the chief technologists of CT and MR, Susan Pogson and Jeanette Rainford, respectively, in their efforts to help with this project. We also wish to thank Tony Ng for his untiring efforts in performing the sinus CT examinations in the evenings. We would like to extend our special appreciation and recognition to our photographer, Roger Harris, for his skills and excellent reproduction of the illustrations and diagrams. We thank Irene Schwerk for her enthusiastic support with some of the illustrations.

The authors wish to acknowledge also the contributors of important illustrative material: M Rontal, E Rontal, E Kassel, W Kuscharczyk, M Chui, D Kirkpatrick and J Cairnes.

We are forever grateful to our spouses and children for letting us have the weekends to be preoccupied with our book. We thank Dr David Hynes, Chief of Diagnostic Imaging, for the encouragement and support he has shown. Last but not least, the authors thank their editor at Martin Dunitz Publishers, Robert Peden, and his assistants who have worked diligently to compile this atlas.

Work for this book was supported by the Research Foundation of St Joseph's Health Centre, Toronto, Canada.

The research for Chapter 5 was supported by the Saul A. Silverman Family Foundation and the Latner Family Trust as a Canada-International Scientific Exchange Program in Otolaryngology (CISEPO II) Project.

For Chapter 13 three-dimensional reconstructions were performed by Dr Lofchy using VI hardware and software contained within the ALLEGRO medical imaging workstation (ISG Technologies Inc., Toronto) in co-operation with the Volume Investigation Laboratory, The Toronto Hospital, Toronto Western Division, University of Toronto.

Chapter 15 is based on an article forthcoming in the *Journal of Otolaryngology*, with the kind permission of the editor.

Figures 1.1, 2.3, 2.4 and 3.17–3.19 are reproduced from H Stammberger, *Functional endoscopic sinus surgery: The Messerklinger technique* (St Louis: Mosby-YearBook 1991) by kind permission of the publisher.

Figures 3.10–3.16 and 3.20–3.22 are reproduced from M Rontal, E Rontal, 'Studying whole-mounted sections of the paranasal sinuses to understand the complications of endoscopic sinus surgery', *The Laryngoscope* (1991) 101: 361–6, by kind permission of the editor and the authors.

Figure 5.6 is used by courtesy of Dr E Kasel, SBK.

Figure 8.16 is used by courtesy of Dr J Cairnes and Dr D Kirkpatrick, Dalhousie University, Halifax.

Figures 8.28, 9.18, 9.28 and 12.52 are used by courtesy of Dr M Chui, St Michael's Hospital, Toronto.

Figures 12.35, 12.36, 12.47–12.50 and 12.53–12.62 are used by courtesy of Dr W Kuscharczyk, Tri-Hospital MR Centre, Toronto.

LS
MH
KE
HS

1

Introduction to functional endoscopic sinus surgery

The concept of functional endoscopic sinus surgery was developed by Professor Walter Messerklinger in Graz, Austria, in the early 1970s following extensive research into the pathophysiology and anatomy of the paranasal sinuses. Messerklinger's concepts have revolutionized, improved and radically altered the techniques used for the diagnosis and treatment of patients with sinus disease. The concepts of functional endoscopic sinus surgery were popularized and exported from the German-speaking countries by Heinz Stammberger in 1984 and David Kennedy in 1985.

Endoscopic sinus surgery evolved from a combination of the techniques of intranasal surgery, which originated in the nineteenth century, and from endoscopy of the lateral nasal wall, a technique that was initially used only as a diagnostic tool.

Intranasal surgery to facilitate the drainage of purulent secretions was initially reported in the late nineteenth century. Inferior meatal antrostomy (fenestration) was described in the late 1890s and middle meatal antrostomy in 1886 by Mikulicz and again in 1899 by Siebenmann. At that time it was noted that middle meatal antrostomies did not stenose with the same rapidity as did those performed in the inferior meatus; however, the surgeons of those pre-antibiotic times were deterred by the close anatomic relationship of the orbit to the site of the middle meatal antrostomy.

Inflammatory disease of the paranasal sinuses requiring surgery has until recently been treated surgically with radical procedures such as the Caldwell–Luc radical antrostomy, intranasal ethmoidectomy and external frontoethmoidectomy. All of these radical surgical procedures involve the extensive removal of diseased mucosa. While these procedures should not be totally excluded from the list of available surgical options for the treatment of benign sinus disease, the majority of patients with chronic sinusitis are more appropriately treated with the minimally invasive and more conservative technique of functional endoscopic sinus surgery.

Hilding, in 1944, elegantly demonstrated in animals that there were definite pathways along which the cilia transported and cleared the mucus produced within a sinus, and that the mucus would inevitably pass to and through the natural ostium despite the presence of an inferior meatal intranasal antrostomy, which would be circumnavigated. The importance of this work was not realized at the time and intranasal antrostomies and Caldwell–Luc procedures remained the mainstay of surgical treatment.

Messerklinger's research established that the health of the frontal and the maxillary sinuses is subordinate to the anterior ethmoid, as these sinuses are ventilated from and drain into the nasal cavity via their prechambers (the frontal recess at the entrance to the frontal sinus and the ethmoid infundibulum at the entrance to the maxillary sinus) which connect their ostia to the middle meatus. He also demonstrated that occlusion of the narrow and stenotic clefts (prechambers) of the ethmoid labyrinth, which connect the ostia of the frontal and maxillary sinuses to the anterior ethmoid led to disordered ventilation and decreased mucociliary clearance from the larger (the frontal and maxillary) paranasal sinuses and therefore predisposed the patient to recurrent infections in these larger sinuses.

Messerklinger noted that infection of these larger sinuses was usually rhinogenic in origin, spreading from the nose through the anterior ethmoid to involve the frontal and maxillary sinuses secondarily. He also demonstrated that, despite the fact that the symptoms of infection in these larger sinuses were usually clinically dominant, the underlying cause was generally not to be found in the larger sinuses themselves, but instead in the clefts of the anterior ethmoid in the lateral nasal wall (Figure 1.1). Messerklinger observed that, when infections in the frontal and maxillary sinuses did not heal or recurred promptly, a focus of infection usually persisted in one of the narrow clefts of the anterior ethmoid, with the focus of infection interfering with normal ventilation and drainage of the sinuses, the infection spreading locally to involve the prechambers and secondarily the larger sinuses.

Messerklinger also noted that after a limited endoscopic resection of the disease within the anterior ethmoid that was responsible for the obstruction of the ventilation and drainage pathways of the larger paranasal sinuses, and the re-establishment of drainage and ventilation through the natural pathways, even massive mucosal pathology within the frontal and maxillary sinuses usually healed without direct surgical intervention into these larger sinuses (Figure 1.1). Mucosal changes within the frontal and maxillary sinuses that had previously been regarded as irreversible returned to normal several weeks following what was essentially a minimal, endoscopically controlled resection of disease.

In summary, the key theory of functional endoscopic sinus surgery is that by removing localized disease obstructing the narrow ethmoidal clefts, and thereby restoring normal mucociliary drainage and ventilation, spontaneous resolution of the mucosal disease in the maxillary and frontal sinuses will follow without the need for radical mucosal excision.

Developments in both the design of diagnostic endoscopes and the re-evaluation of radiographic imaging have been instrumental in the evolution of these endoscopic surgical techniques. Hirschmann first described endoscopy of the nasal cavities in 1903. He used an instrument that was designed as a cystoscope. There were many subsequent attempts by a variety of rhinologists to develop a more sophisticated instrument. The development of the operating microscope in the early 1950s improved the intraoperative view of the nasal cavity, especially that of the posterior ethmoid and sphenoid sinuses. The main disadvantage to the microscope was its straight visual field which did not permit an adequate view into the ethmoid clefts. The development of fiberoptic rod telescopes by Hopkins in the late 1950s was a dramatic advance. This optical system includes a light source distant from the instrument and a quartz-rod air-lens system that provides excellent resolution with high contrast and, despite the small diameter of the endoscope, a wide field of vision. With the addition of angled lenses, these endoscopes have made it possible to examine in detail the clefts and recesses of the nasal cavity (Figures 1.2–1.4). Initially, they were used only for diagnostic purposes; however, Messerklinger showed that it was possible to introduce appropriately designed instruments alongside the endoscopes to perform a precise surgical resection under direct vision.

The precise surgical techniques aimed at restoring normal physiological conditions and the preservation of as much mucosa as possible have only developed with the additional anatomic and pathophysiologic information that has been provided by radiographic imaging. Indeed, functional endoscopic sinus surgery has only been developed to its current level because of the advances that have occurred in the fields of radiology.

Messerklinger's initial work in Graz was conducted with information derived from conventional tomographs. This technique has now been superseded by computed tomography (CT) and such imaging is now considered an essential component of the diagnostic investigation of patients presenting with symptoms suggestive of benign inflammatory disease of the paranasal sinuses. CT is the ideal method for the demonstration of the delicate bony leaflets of the ethmoid labyrinth. It also identifies those anatomic variants that may compromise the ventilation of the sinuses, and it can demonstrate those discrete areas of diseased mucosa that are responsible for recurrent disease in the larger paranasal sinuses (the frontal and the maxillary sinuses). The majority of these latter abnormalities will not be evident on even careful diagnostic endoscopic assessment. Because the rhinologist is interested in the detail of the fine structures within the lateral wall of the nose, the radiologists will have to direct their focus towards the drainage pathways and prechambers of the larger paranasal sinuses and away from the obvious abnormalities that may be secondarily present in the larger paranasal sinuses.

CT is now regarded as essential when the patient has undergone previous sinus surgery. In this situation, the scans will provide valuable information about the presence of potential hazards such as dehiscence of the lamina papyracea, the proximity of the orbit to areas of disease, or septation of the frontal or sphenoid sinuses, and about the location of the internal carotid artery and optic nerve. Other important variations, such as a low-lying ethmoid fovea and cribriform plate, and adhesions of the uncinate process to the medial orbital wall, will be discussed in subsequent chapters.

A systematic endoscopic assessment of the lateral nasal wall in conjunction with CT of the nose and paranasal sinuses allows the precise localization of the underlying disease processes and thus aids the clinician in planning the appropriate therapy. The ability to radiologically identify those abnormalities that may increase surgical morbidity prior to commencing the surgical dissection is important both for the surgeon and the patient.

Understandably, there is considerable interest amongst both radiologists and rhinologists in the radiologic anatomy of the paranasal region. Until recently, knowledge of the required radiographic techniques, anatomy and significant pathology of the structures identified by CT has not been included in the curriculum of most radiologists.

The aim of this book is to provide a simple concise atlas to introduce both rhinologists and radiologists to the essential concepts of functional endoscopic sinus surgery, and to point out the relevant anatomy and, in particular, the anatomic variants that may predispose the patient to recurrent sinusitis. This information is important to both surgeons and radiologists so that the CT scans can be interpreted prior to and at the time of surgery.

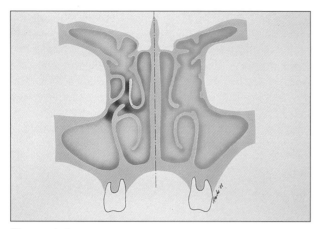

Figure **1.1**

This schematic drawing demonstrates the key diseased area of the anterior ethmoid on the left. The situation after functional endoscopic sinus surgery is shown on the right.

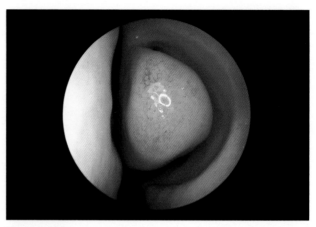

Figure **1.2**

Concha bullosa: endoscopic view. The grossly widened left middle tubinate contained a single large air cell. This type of middle turbinate is known as a concha bullosa.

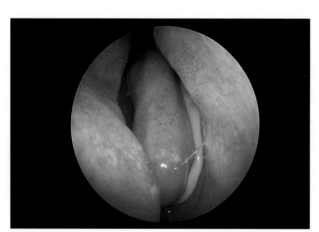

Figure **1.3**

Chronic sinusitis: endoscopic view. This patient presented with left-sided chronic maxillary sinusitis. Note the creamy white purulent material draining from the left semilunar hiatus.

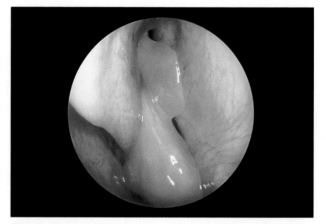

Figure **1.4**

Nasal polyps: endoscopic view. Several yellowish nasal polyps can be seen arising from the right middle meatus.

2

Nasal physiology

The nose and paranasal sinuses have multiple functions that include the provision of an upper respiratory air channel, filtering and humidification of inspired air, olfaction, vocal resonance, speech and nasal reflex functions. For the purpose of this text, attention will only be drawn towards those functions which are of significance in the pathogenesis of sinusitis, or in the interpretation of sinus radiographs and computed tomographs (CT) of the paranasal sinuses.

The nose and paranasal sinuses are lined with a ciliated, pseudostratified columnar epithelium, beneath which lies the tunica propria, containing serous and mucous glands. The main function of the nose is to transmit, filter, warm and humidify the inspired air. The two most important factors contributing to the maintenance of the normal physiology of the paranasal sinuses and their lining of mucous membranes are drainage and ventilation. Normal drainage of the paranasal sinuses requires a complex balance between the production of mucous and its transportation through and out of the sinus. This balance is to a large extent dependent upon the amount of mucus produced within the sinus, and its composition and viscosity, the effectiveness of the ciliary beat, mucosal reabsorption and the condition of the ostia and the ethmoid clefts through which the mucus must pass on its way into the nasal cavity. Ventilation and drainage of the frontal and maxillary sinuses depend primarily upon the patency of both the actual sinus ostia and their ethmoid prechambers, which connect the ostia with the nasal cavity via the anterior ethmoid.

SECRETION OF MUCUS

Under normal conditions the mucous blanket that covers and protects the nasal mucosa is continuously produced by the mucoserous nasal glands and the intraepithelial goblet cells. The mucous blanket has two layers, an inner serous layer which is called the sol phase in which the cilia beat, and an outer more viscous layer, the gel phase which is transported on top of the sol phase by the ciliary beat. The balance between the underlying sol phase and the outer gel phase is critically important for the maintenance of normal mucociliary clearance. Under normal conditions dust and other fine particles become incorporated into the gel phase and are transported with the mucus out of the sinuses. The mucous layer is continuously produced and steadily transported away from the sinus. A healthy maxillary sinus renews its mucous layer on average every 20 to 30 minutes.

VENTILATION AND DRAINAGE

The ostia of the two largest and clinically most important sinuses, the frontal and the maxillary sinuses, communicate with the middle meatus by very narrow and delicate 'prechambers'. The frontal sinus opens into an hour-glass shaped cleft, the frontal recess (Figure 2.3). The maxillary sinus ostium opens into a cleft in the lateral nasal wall, the ethmoid infundibulum (Figure 2.4). Both of these clefts or prechambers (the frontal recess and the infundibulum) are part of the anterior ethmoid complex. If these prechambers become obstructed, then the drainage and ventilation of the frontal and maxillary sinuses will be impaired, and a secondary infection within these sinuses is likely to develop.

The nasal mucosa is innervated by the autonomic nervous system, with parasympathetic stimulation causing an increased serous type of secretion and sympathetic stimulation causing an increased mucinous secretion.

NASAL BLOOD FLOW AND SUPPLY

The nasal mucosa has an abundant blood flow which is derived from both the internal and the external carotid arterial systems. The main arterial supply is derived from the sphenopalatine branch of the maxillary artery, as well as contributions from the anterior and posterior ethmoidal branches of the ophthalmic artery.

Special areas of erectile cavernous tissue overlie the inferior turbinate and the inferior margin and posterior end of the middle turbinate. Similar tissue may also be present in the submucosa of the nasal septum anteriorly, where it is known variously as the 'septal swell body', the 'tuberculum septi' or as the 'tumescence of Zuckerkandl' (Figure 2.1).

The autonomic nerve supply of the blood vessels is derived from the superior cervical sympathetic ganglion and from the sphenopalatine ganglion, which relays the parasympathetic nerve fibers. Sympathetic stimulation causes vasoconstriction and parasympathetic stimulation causes vasodilatation. Blood flow can be affected by a variety of local factors, including temperature, humidity, trauma and infection, as well as by the administration of vasodilator or vasoconstrictor drugs. Blood flow is also altered by hormonal change, i.e. hyper- and hypothyroidism, as well as by estrogens being raised during menstruation and pregnancy. Emotional stress may cause either vasoconstriction or vasodilatation.

Our experience with the administration of topical nasal decongestants prior to CT examination demonstrated several changes in the nasal mucosa following the administration of 0.1% xylometazoline hydrochloride nasal solution (Figures 2.2, 2.5). There was shrinking of the inferior turbinates and of the nasal swell body. The middle turbinates and the ethmoidal prechambers remained unaffected.

The extent of vasodilatation (thickness) of the nasal mucosa has a great effect upon the resistance of the nasal airway. Vasodilatation is dependent both on the autonomic control of the blood flow and on the nasal cycle.

The erectile tissue of the nasal cavity is also affected by postural changes. For example, when lying on one's side in bed, the mucosa of the dependent nasal cavity slowly undergoes engorgement as blood pools in the venous sinusoids under the effect of gravity.

THE NASAL CYCLE

The nasal cycle is the term used to describe the normal paradoxical opening and closing of alternate sides of the nasal airway. This normally alternates from side to side approximately every 2–3 hours. The factors controlling the nasal cycle are at present unknown (Figure 2.6).

Zinreich and Kennedy (1988c) have demonstrated the cyclical changes of the nasal cycle in normal volunteers using magnetic resonance imaging. On T2-weighted scans, the increase in signal intensity and mucosal volume was seen to be limited to the turbinates (inferior and middle), the ethmoidal prechambers and the nasal septum. These changes alternated from side to side over the course of the day. This increased signal intensity is indistinguishable from inflamed mucosa. To define the extent of inflammation separate from the normal nasal cycle, topical decongestants can be administered. This results in a prompt reversal of the nasal cycle. Malignancy, such as squamous cell carcinoma, has a low signal intensity relative to brain on T2-weighted images, so that it can be easily differentiated from the normal nasal cycle and from inflamed mucosa.

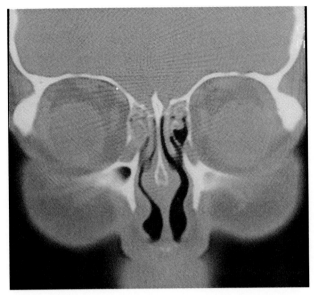

2.1

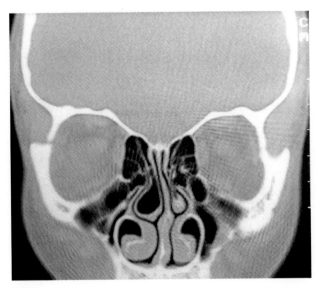

2.2A

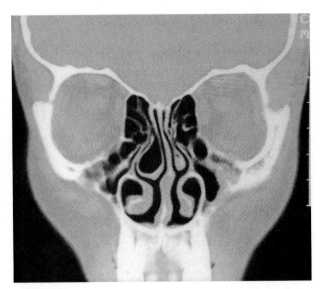

2.2B

Figure **2.1**

The septal swell body. The bulbous swelling on the anterior nasal septum in this coronal CT scan is produced by an area of submucosal erectile tissue known variously as the nasal septal swell body, the tuberculum septi and the tumescence of Zuckerkandl.

Figure **2.2**

The effects of topical decongestants. The effect of a topical nasal decongestant upon the nasal mucous membranes is illustrated in this pair of photographs. The coronal CT scan seen in A was taken prior to the administration of a 0.1% solution of xylometazoline. Note, in B, the vasoconstriction of the inferior turbinates 10 minutes after the application of the topical nasal decongestant solution.

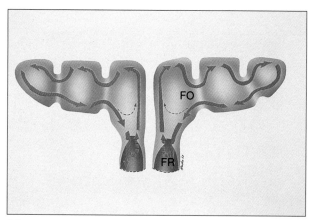

2.3

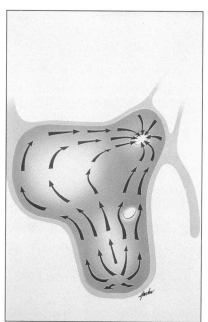

2.4A

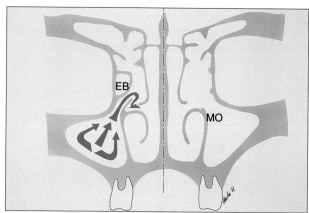

2.4B

Figure **2.3**

This schematic drawing shows the normal mucociliary
transportation route inside and out of the frontal sinuses. FO,
the frontal sinus ostium; FR, the frontal recess, which is the
ethmoid prechamber which connects the frontal sinus ostium to
the anterior ethmoid. (After Stammberger, 1991.)

Figure **2.4**

These schematic drawings show the normal transportation
pathways of mucus inside (A) and moving out of (B) a maxillary
sinus. EB, the ethmoid bulla; MO, the maxillary sinus ostium.
Note the infundibulum, the prechamber which connects the
maxillary sinus ostium with the nasal cavity via the semilunar
hiatus. The infundibulum is the space lying between the
uncinate process and the ethmoid bulla. (After Stammberger,
1991.)

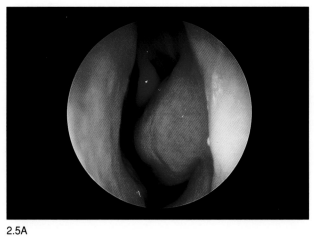

2.5A

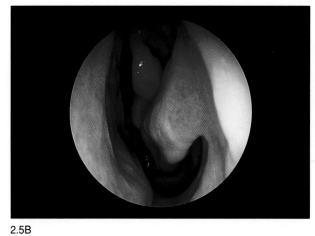

2.5B

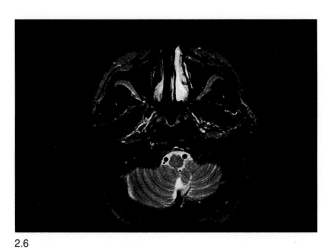

2.6

Figure 2.5

The effects of topical decongestants: endoscopic view. The submucosal layer of the inferior turbinates contains large areas of erectile tissue. The view in A is of a normal left inferior turbinate: the anterior end of the left middle turbinate can just be seen above and posterior to the inferior turbinate. The same inferior turbinate is seen in B 10 minutes after the application of a topical nasal decongestant. The inferior turbinate is much smaller and the anterior end of the middle turbinate is more readily seen.

Figure 2.6

The nasal cycle. The engorgement and vasodilatation of the left inferior turbinate from the normal nasal cycle is seen in this T2-weighted MR scan as a hyperintense (white) area.

3

Gross and sectional anatomy of the nasal cavity and paranasal sinuses

The nasal cavity is a midline structure extending from the base of the skull to the roof of the mouth. It is divided in the midline by the nasal septum into two symmetrical nasal fossae (Figure 3.1). The nasal cavity communicates anteriorly through the nares with the exterior and posteriorly through the posterior choanae with the nasopharynx. The nasal cavity also communicates through the lateral nasal wall with the maxillary and frontal sinuses, and more posteriorly with the sphenoid sinuses.

The roof of the nasal cavity is formed by the nasal and frontal bones anteriorly; the cribriform plate of the ethmoid bone in the middle; and the sphenoid, alae of the vomer and the sphenoidal process of the palatine bone posteriorly. The cribriform plate, which is only 2–3 mm wide, is perforated by approximately 20 foramina which transmit fibers of the olfactory nerve. The thin lateral lamina of the cribriform plate is the most vulnerable area surgically (Figure 3.2).

The floor of the nasal cavity is formed by the bones of the hard palate, namely the palatine process of the maxilla anteriorly and the horizontal plate of the palatine bone posteriorly.

The medial wall of each nasal cavity is formed by the nasal septum which passes from the roof of the cavity to the floor. The nasal septum is partly bony and partly cartilaginous. The anterior attachment of the cartilaginous septum is with the upper and lower lateral nasal cartilages superiorly, and the maxillary crest inferiorly. An accessory cartilage of Huschke may lie along this latter articulation and narrow the nasal cavity. The bony septum is composed of the perpendicular plate of the ethmoid superiorly and the vomer posteroinferiorly. The bony septum is attached posteriorly to the body of the sphenoid and anteriorly to both the nasal bones and the spine of the frontal bone.

Up to 25% of the population have some deviation of the nasal septum. These deviations may occur in either the cartilaginous septum, the bony septum or in both parts. The nasal septal cartilage may be dislocated from the maxillary crest. Such deviations may be due to asymmetrical growth or trauma, either during parturition or at a later date. There is not infrequently an apparent thickening of the cartilaginous nasal septum in its upper third, known as the tuberculum septi or nasal septal swell body, described by Zuckerkandl. This is caused by an area of rudimentary erectile tissue found on each side of the septum. This swell body often overlies a thickening of the bony septum.

The lateral wall of the nasal cavity can be divided into three parts. Anteriorly the lateral nasal wall consists of the frontal process of the maxilla and the lacrimal bone. The middle portion is formed by the ethmoid labyrinth, the maxilla and the inferior turbinate. The posterior portion of the lateral nasal wall is formed by the perpendicular plate of the palatine bone and the medial pterygoid plate of the sphenoid. Protruding from the lateral wall are three shelf-like structures, the superior, middle and inferior turbinates with their corresponding meatus inferolaterally. The lateral wall of the nasal cavity (Figures 3.3–3.5) will be discussed in greater detail later.

Anteriorly the nasal cavity communicates with the exterior through the piriform aperture of the maxilla, the nasal bones and the cartilage comprising the external nose.

Posteriorly the nasal cavity communicates with the nasopharynx through the choanae. These are bounded superiorly by the body of the sphenoid and the alae of the vomer; inferiorly by the posterior border of the horizontal process of the palatine bone and soft palate; laterally by the medial pterygoid plate of the sphenoid bone and medially by the posterior border of the vomer.

THE INFERIOR TURBINATE AND THE INFERIOR MEATUS

The inferior turbinate is a thin curved lamina which attaches to the nasal surface of the maxilla and the perpendicular plate of the palatine bone. Its lower free border is gently curved. Three bony prominences project from the superior free border of the inferior turbinate. The most anterior is the lacrimal process, which attaches to the lacrimal bone and the nasolacrimal groove of the maxilla, thereby helping to form the medial wall of the nasolacrimal duct. The ethmoidal process of the inferior turbinate is attached to the uncinate process and separates the anterior fontanelle from the posterior fontanelle. The third prominence, the maxillary process, projects inferiorly and laterally to attach on to the maxilla and the maxillary process of the palatine bone, thus forming part of the medial wall of the maxillary sinus. Inferolateral to the inferior turbinate lies the inferior meatus, which is deepest at the junction of its anterior and middle thirds. The nasolacrimal duct open into this part of this meatus and is protected by Hasner's valve (Figure 3.6).

THE PTERYGOPALATINE FOSSA

The pterygopalatine fossa is an inverted pyramidal space located between the posterior surface of the maxillary sinus and the anterior surface of the pterygoid plates. The pterygopalatine fossa should not be mistaken for the pterygoid fossa which lies between medial and lateral pterygoid plates. The principle contents of the pterygopalatine fossa are the sphenopalatine ganglion, the maxillary nerve, and the maxillary artery and its accompanying veins. The sphenopalatine ganglion relays the parasympathetic nerve supply to the lacrimal gland, the mucous glands of the nose, nasopharynx and paranasal sinuses, and the palate. The maxillary nerve is the second division of the trigeminal nerve, which supplies sensation to the middle third of the face.

The pterygopalatine fossa connects through fissures and foramina with several important spaces (Figure 3.7): laterally, with the infratemporal fossa through the pterygomaxillary fissure; anteriorly, to the orbit through the infraorbital fissure; posteriorly, to the middle cranial fossa through the foramen rotundum and the pterygoid canal; medially, to the

inferior portion of the sphenoethmoid recess through the sphenopalatine foramen and the oral cavity through the greater and lesser palatine foramina.

GROSS ANATOMY OF THE PARANASAL SINUSES

The paranasal sinuses consist of the maxillary, the ethmoid, frontal and sphenoid sinuses. The anatomy of each sinus is variable, but it is the anatomy of the ethmoid bone and its attendant air cells that is the most challenging to comprehend. Understanding the anatomy of the middle meatus and lateral nasal wall is paramount for the practising surgeon using sinus endoscopy.

The frontal sinus

The frontal bone is one of the unpaired skull bones forming the anterior portion of the calvarium. The frontal bone articulates with the ethmoid, the sphenoid, the parietal and the nasal bones, as well as with the zygoma and the maxilla. The frontal bone is occasionally divided in the midline by a persistent metopic suture. The frontal bone contains marrow, and consequently, it is susceptible to osteomyelitis. The frontal bone makes a major contribution to the floor of the anterior cranial fossa and in so doing forms the roof of the orbits (Figure 3.6). The inferior surface of the frontal bone is notched by the ethmoid foveolae which close the open roof of the ethmoid labyrinths (Figure 3.8).

The frontal sinus is undeveloped at birth, appearing in the second year as an outgrowth of the frontal recess. On average, the top of the frontal sinus lies at the level of the midvertical height of the orbit by the age of 4 years and reaches the height of the supraorbital rim by 8 years. It extends above the orbit by 10 years of age. The frontal sinus extends superiorly into the superciliary region and posteriorly above the medial part of the roof of the orbit. The two frontal sinuses are usually unequal in size and separated by a bony septum which does not lie in the midline. There may be numerous incomplete septa giving the sinus its characteristic scalloped outline. Secretions from the frontal sinus drain through the frontal recess into the middle meatus (Figure 3.21).

The thin posterior wall of the frontal sinus overlies the dura of the anterior cranial fossa, and, consequently, infections within the frontal sinus can spread through its posterior wall, resulting in an extradural abscess.

The maxillary sinus

The maxilla consists of a body and several processes: the zygomatic, frontal, palatine and alveolar processes. The maxilla attaches to the frontal bone, the palatine bone, the zygoma, the ethmoid, the nasal bone and with the lacrimal bones.

The maxillary sinus is a space within the body of the maxilla which is usually present at birth as a slit-like cavity. Normally, this rudimentary maxillary sinus extends under the infraorbital canal by 2 years and into the zygoma by 9 years of age.

The maxillary sinus is pyramidal in shape, with the base forming the medial wall of the sinus and the apex pointing into the zygomatic process of the maxilla. In some instances, the maxillary sinus may be compartmentalized by usually incomplete bony septa. The anterior and posterior walls of the maxillary sinus consist of the anterior and posterior walls of the maxilla. The roof of the maxillary sinus is the floor of the orbit, which exhibits a ridge occupied by the infraorbital nerve. The floor of the maxillary sinus is formed by the alveolar recess, which lies at a lower level than the floor of the nasal cavity. This area bears upon the upper teeth, with the roots of the first molar and the second premolar lying in close proximity to the floor of the sinus. Later in life these roots may project through the floor, although they are still usually covered by a thin layer of bone and mucosa. Superomedially, the ethmomaxillary plate separates the maxillary sinus from the posterior ethmoid air cells (Figure 3.13).

The bony medial wall of the maxillary sinus is deficient in two areas. These areas, which are closed by periosteum and mucous membrane, are the anterior and the posterior nasal fontanelles. The ostium of the maxillary sinus opens into the depth of the ethmoid infundibulum at a point approximately transecting the midpoint between the anterior and posterior insertions of the inferior turbinate. Accessory maxillary sinus ostia are frequently found in both the anterior and the posterior fontanelles. When present, these accessory maxillary sinus ostia can usually be seen on diagnostic endoscopy, whereas the true maxillary ostium cannot usually be seen as it remains concealed by the uncinate process (Figures 3.3 and 3.14).

The sphenoid sinus

The sphenoid bone is another of the unpaired skull bones (Figures 3.7 and 3.9). The sphenoid bone consists of a body that gives origin to the lesser wings superiorly, and the greater wings and pterygoid processes inferiorly. It attaches to the basi-occiput, the petrous and the squamous temporal bones, the parietal bone, the frontal bone, the vomer and the perpendicular plate of the palatine bone. The sphenoid bone is traversed by the foramen rotundum, the foramen ovale, the pterygoid canal (vidian canal), the optic canal and the superior orbital fissure.

The sphenoid sinus lies within the body of the sphenoid bone. The front of the body of the sphenoid bone is ridged by the rostrum which articulates with the perpendicular plate of the ethmoid and the nasal septum. This ridge projects into the sinus as the intersinus septum which rarely lies in the midline. The sphenoid sinus is barely present at birth, and its subsequent pneumatization is both variable and asymmetrical. The sphenoid sinus may lie solely anterior to the pituitary fossa and gland, or it may extend posteriorly into the basiocciput and laterally into the roots of the pterygoid process. The floor of the sphenoid sinus may be ridged by the pterygoid canal transmitting the vidian nerve. The sphenoid sinus ostia, which are located on the anterior wall of the sinus, open into the spheno-ethmoidal recess which is located posterior to the superior turbinate (Figures 3.4–3.6 and 3.21).

The optic nerve has an intimate relationship with the internal carotid artery. The internal carotid artery courses through the petrous temporal bone to emerge medially at the petrous apex above the foramen lacerum (Figures 3.11 and 3.12). It deeply grooves the body of the sphenoid in an S-shape before turning back upon itself medial to the anterior clinoid process. Above the body of the sphenoid lies the pituitary fossa, containing the pituitary gland surrounded by the cavernous sinus. The optic chiasma lies above the pituitary gland. From it extends the two optic nerves, surrounded by the meninges and accompanied by the ophthalmic arteries as they pass through the optic canals.

The ethmoid sinuses

The ethmoid bone contributes to the medial wall of the orbit, the nasal septum, the floor of the anterior cranial fossa and the lateral wall of the nasal cavity. It is another of the unpaired skull bones and is composed of five parts: a perpendicular plate (which comprises a portion of the bony nasal septum), a horizontal plate (the cribriform plate), a superior prominence (the crista galli), and two multicellular labyrinths, containing the anterior and posterior ethmoid air cells, suspended laterally. The ethmoid labyrinths are narrow anteriorly and expend as they pass posteriorly and follow the natural lateral curve of the medial wall of the orbit (Figure 3.2).

The anatomy of the ethmoid labyrinths is initially challenging. These bony chambers are enclosed by the ethmoid bone in the lateral and medial planes only. Anteriorly the cells are closed by the lacrimal bone laterally. Superiorly the labyrinthine cells are closed by the indentations in the thicker inferior surface of the frontal bone known as the ethmoid foveolae. The posterior ethmoid air cells are closed by the anterolateral walls of the sphenoid sinus (Figure 3.22).

The lateral bony plate of the ethmoid, which is named the lamina papyracea, forms the medial wall of the orbit. The lamina papyracea is extremely thin and it may be dehiscent in part, allowing disease to track through into the orbit (Figure 3.11). The medial wall of the ethmoid labyrinth is composed of the middle turbinate, the superior turbinate and, when present, the supreme turbinate. Inferior and lateral to the middle turbinate is a cleft known as the middle meatus, and inferolateral to the superior turbinate is the superior meatus (Figures 3.14 and 3.15). The ethmoid clefts open medially into the nasal cavity and posteriorly into the choanae. The spheno-ethmoidal recess is located posterosuperior to the superior turbinate (Figure 3.13).

The ethmoid air cells are divided into an anterior and a posterior group. The anterior ethmoid air cells drain into the middle meatus, whereas the posterior ethmoid air cells drain into the superior meatus. The largest and most constant anterior ethmoid air cell is named the ethmoid bulla and the most anterior of these cells are the agger nasi cells (both the ethmoid bulla and the agger nasi cells will be discussed in more detail later) (Figures 3.16 and 3.20). The most posterior ethmoid air cells are called Onodi's cells (cells of Onodi). They may extend posterolaterally to embrace or even surround the optic nerve (Figure 3.12). These cells may migrate into the body of the sphenoid and even reach the anterior wall of the sella turcica.

Medial to the vertical insertion of the middle turbinate lies the cribriform plate through which the olfactory nerve fibers pass (Figure 3.2). The cribriform plate lies at a lower level than the roofs of the adjacent ethmoid air cells and tends to dip inferiorly as it passes posteriorly. The attendant dura, olfactory bulb and frontal lobe should always be considered to be at risk during ethmoidal surgery. Injury to the cribriform plate may cause a cerebrospinal fluid leak and/or permanent anosmia. Behind the cribriform plate the nasal cavity is roofed by the thicker horizontal plate of sphenoid bone, the planum spenoidale.

The agger nasi

The agger nasi (the agger mound) is a smooth bony swelling or eminence in the frontal process of the maxilla; it lies in front of the anterior insertion of the middle turbinate (Figures 3.6 and 3.16). The agger nasi may be pneumatized in a variable manner by the agger nasi air cells of the anterior ethmoid, and its bony wall may therefore be either thick or thin. Both the lacrimal sac and the frontal recess lie lateral to the agger nasi when the agger is not pneumatized. Anterolateral to the agger nasi and running parallel to it is the nasolacrimal duct. The frontal recess the nasolacrimal duct and the agger nasi all lie in a similar coronal plane.

The middle turbinate and the ground lamella

The middle turbinate is an integral part of the ethmoid bone. It has a vertical, anterior free border that may be slender or bulbous. Occasionally this free border is lobulated. The posterior margin is attached to the lateral nasal wall and to the perpendicular plate of the palatine bone. Immediately posterior to this attachment lies the sphenopalatine foramen transmitting the sphenopalatine vessels and the posterior superior nasal nerves. The middle turbinate may be pneumatized in both the anterior or the posterior segments. Such a middle turbinate air cell is called a 'concha bullosa'.

The middle turbinate (Figure 3.10) attaches to the skull base and to the lateral wall of the nasal cavity in a diverse manner. This attachment can be divided into three parts.

i   The anterior portion of the middle turbinate lies in a paramedian sagittal plane. The vertical lamella of the middle turbinate inserts into the lateral border of the cribriform plate and is covered medially by olfactory epithelium containing fibers of the olfactory nerve in the superior portion. Careless dissection leading to avulsion of this medial lamella may lead to leakage of cerebrospinal fluid and the risk of intracranial sepsis (Figure 3.14).

ii   The vertical plate of the central portion of the middle turbinate rotates to lie in the coronal plane between the anterior portion medially and the lamina papyracea laterally. This part is known as the ground or basal lamella of the middle turbinate. This lamella is anatomically important because it divides the anterior ethmoid air cells from the posterior ethmoid air cells. All of the air cells anterior to the ground lamella have their ostia located in the anterior ethmoid, whereas all of the ethmoid air cells posterior to the ground lamella have their ostia located in the superior meatus. The sphenoid sinus ostia open into the sphenoethmoid recess (Figure 3.15).

iii   The posterior portion of the insertion of the middle turbinate runs in a horizontal plane forming the roof of the posterior middle meatus. The bone inserts into the lamina papyracea or medial wall of the maxilla.

The lateral wall of the middle meatus houses several key anatomic features (Figures 3.3, 3.4, 3.6, 3.14 and 3.21). These are the uncinate process, semilunar hiatus, ethmoid infundibulum, ethmoid bulla, lateral sinus and frontal recess.

The uncinate process

The uncinate process is a fine bony leaflet which lies immediately posterior to the agger nasi. This thin bony prominence is usually found posterior to the leading vertical edge of the middle turbinate on the lateral wall of the nasal cavity. It can be exposed by gentle medial retraction of the middle turbinate. The superior origin of the uncinate process from the lateral bony nasal wall is variable. It may insert into the lamina papyracea, the lacrimal bone or the skull base, and it may even swing medially to insert into the lateral surface of the middle turbinate (Figures 3.14, 3.19 and 3.21). Its upper extremity is usually concealed by the anterior insertion of the middle turbinate. The uncinate process then sweeps down in a posteroinferior direction, curving more posteri-

orly in its lower portion. The uncinate process forms the medial wall of the infundibulum, and its posterior free margin forms the anterior boundary of the semilunar hiatus.

At the posterior inferior insertion of the uncinate process, fine bony spicules attach the uncinate process to the perpendicular plate of the palatine bone. Further bony spicules arise from the inferior margin of the uncinate process and articulate with the ethmoid process of the inferior turbinate. It is this latter bony attachment that separates the anterior and posterior fontanelles. These are bony defects, of variable size, in the medial wall of the maxillary sinus; they are covered by mucoperiosteum and transmit the accessory maxillary ostia when they are present.

The semilunar hiatus

The semilunar hiatus is a two-dimensional cleft that lies between the posterior free margin of the uncinate process and the anterior wall of the ethmoid bulla. It is usually 1–2 mm wide and forms the entrance into the ethmoid infundibulum, which lies lateral to the uncinate process (Figure 3.4).

The ethmoid infundibulum

The ethmoid infundibulum is a three-dimensional space lying lateral to the uncinate process. The medial wall of the infundibulum is formed by the uncinate process, whereas its lateral wall is formed by the lamina papyracea with a variable contribution from the frontal process of the maxilla and from the lacrimal bone (Figure 3.20).

The anatomy of the superior part of the infundibulum varies depending on the bony insertion of the uncinate process. If the uncinate process inserts laterally onto the lamina papyracea the infundibulum ends superiorly as a blind pit known as the terminal recess. The frontal sinus drains into the frontal recess which, in this situation, is separated from the infundibulum, thereby limiting the spread of infection from the maxillary sinus to the frontal sinus. If the uncinate process inserts into the roof of the ethmoid, or passes medially to insert into the middle turbinate, the frontal sinus and the frontal recess will open directly into the infundibulum and infection in the maxillary sinus may affect frontal sinus drainage or vice versa.

The infundibulum usually terminates posteriorly at the anterior wall of the ethmoid bulla, where it communicates with the middle meatus via the semilunar hiatus.

The maxillary ostium is hidden deep in the posterior inferior portion of the infundibulum and cannot normally be seen with an endoscope in the middle meatus. However, accessory maxillary ostia may be readily seen perforating the anterior and posterior fontanelles.

Pneumatization of infundibular cells, agger nasi cells or even the uncinate process may occur, distorting the anatomy and sometimes causing the uncinate process to bend medially or even to double back anteriorly.

The lateral margin of the infundibulum is rarely further than 1.0–1.5 mm from the lamina papyracea. It may be further collapsed if there are anatomic variations such as concha bullosa, or pathologic conditions that compress the uncinate process against the lateral nasal wall.

The ethmoid bulla

The ethmoid bulla is the most constant and largest of the anterior ethmoid air cells (Figures 3.3, 3.6 and 3.14). It is pneumatized in a variable manner and, in some individuals, a bony lateral torus is found in the same position. Laterally, the bulla is attached to the lamina papyracea. Posteriorly, it may attach to the ground lamella of the middle turbinate or be separated from it by a posterior extension of the lateral sinus, if present. Superiorly, the bulla may fuse with the roof of the ethmoid and form the posterior wall of the frontal recess, or it may be separated from the ethmoid roof by a space (the lateral sinus) allowing communication between these two spaces.

The lateral sinus

The lateral sinus is a variable cleft found superior and posterior to the ethmoid bulla (Figure 3.18). It lies between the lamina papyracea and the middle turbinate medially. The roof of the ethmoid is found superiorly and the ethmoid bulla inferiorly. Posteriorly, the cleft may be extensive between the bulla and the ground lamella of the middle turbinate. Anteriorly, the lateral sinus may communicate with the frontal recess or it may be separated by the bulla inserting into the roof of the ethmoid.

The frontal recess

The frontal sinus originates from pneumatization of the anterior part of the frontal recess (Figures 3.2 and 3.4). The posterior wall of the frontal recess is variable, depending on the insertion of the ethmoid bulla (Figure 3.19). If the anterior wall of the ethmoid bulla inserts into the roof of the ethmoid, it will form the posterior wall of the frontal recess, thus separating it from the lateral sinus. However, this wall is often incomplete or absent allowing the frontal recess to communicate with the lateral sinus. Depending on the anterosuperior insertion of the uncinate process, the frontal recess may open into the middle meatus or into the ethmoid infundibulum. The frontal recess may be reduced in volume by surrounding structures such as a prominent ethmoid bulla or prominent agger nasi cells.

The frontonasal duct is more appropriately named the frontal recess. It is rarely duct-like and consists instead of a waisted bony recess facilitating ventilation between the frontal sinus and the nasal cavity. The shape of the duct depends mainly on the surrounding structures. The medial border is usually the lateral lamella of the most anterior portion of the middle turbinate. The lateral border consists mainly of lamina papyracea with a small contribution from the uncinate process. Superiorly, the frontal bone forms the roof with its anterior ethmoid foveolae, further anteriorly curving upwards to form the anterior wall of the frontal sinus. The frontal ostium is usually found in the most anterosuperior part of the frontal recess, but this can rarely be seen directly with the endoscope during a routine diagnostic nasal examination (Figure 3.21).

The ostiomeatal complex

The term ostiomeatal complex is used to refer collectively to the maxillary sinus ostia, the ethmoid infundibulum, the semilunar hiatus, the middle meatus, the frontal recess, the ethmoid bulla and the uncinate process. It describes the final common drainage pathways of the frontal, maxillary and anterior ethmoid sinuses.

Haller's cells are ethmoid air cells that invaginate the floor of the orbit in the vicinity of the maxillary sinus ostium. If enlarged, Haller's cells may restrict the ethmoid infundibulum and the ostium of the maxillary sinus. The presence of such a cell usually remains obscured on endoscopic examination of the nasal cavity, however it may be revealed on maxillary sinuscopy and certainly by coronal computed tomography. The origin of these cells is as yet uncertain, but the majority have been noted to open into the middle meatus and therefore are assumed to be of anterior ethmoid origin.

The anterior and posterior ethmoid arteries

The anterior ethmoid artery arises from the ophthalmic artery in the orbit, which in turn arises from the internal carotid artery. It passes through the anterior ethmoid foramen, running obliquely through the frontoethmoid suture, approximately 2–4 mm posterior to the lacrimal crest. The anterior ethmoid artery is surrounded by thin bone and lies above the anterior border of the ethmoid bulla. This bony canal may be embedded in the roof of the ethmoid or connected to it by a bony mesentery. The artery passes through the lateral lamina of the cribriform plate posterior to the crista galli and enters the anterior cranial fossa through the lateral margin of the cribriform plate. It should be noted that this is the thinnest and weakest portion of the skull base. The anterior ethmoid artery supplies the anterior ethmoid air cells and the frontal sinus, and sends intracranial branches to supply the dura. Further terminal branches pass down through the cribriform plate to supply the superior part of the medial and lateral wall of the nasal cavity and a part of the external nose.

The posterior ethmoid artery is also a branch of the ophthalmic artery. It passes through the posterior ethmoidal foramen in the frontoethmoid suture approximately 12 mm posterior to the anterior ethmoid foramen and passes behind the cribriform plate. It also supplies the dura, and further terminal branches pass inferiorly through the cribriform plate to supply the posterosuperior aspects of the lateral and medial nasal wall.

The orbital apex

Structures in the orbital apex are in close proximity to the posterior ethmoid and the sphenoid sinuses, and must be considered at risk from disease or surgery in the vicinity (Figures 3.7, 3.11 and 3.12). The bony orbital apex houses three canals:

i   the optic canal, transmitting the optic nerve and the ophthalmic artery;

ii the superior orbital fissure transmitting the lacrimal, frontal and nasociliary nerves of the ophthalmic division of the trigeminal nerve, and the oculomotor, trochlear and abducent cranial nerves;

iii the inferior orbital fissure transmitting the infraorbital nerve and artery.

A tendinous ring surrounds the medial aspect of the superior orbital fissure and the optic canal. From this ring arise the medial, lateral, superior and inferior recti muscles. Levator palpebrae superioris and the superior oblique muscles arise from bone just superior to the tendinous ring. In this way, the optic nerve and globe are surrounded by a cone of muscle. The lacrimal, frontal and trochlear nerves pass anteriorly within the ring.

The lacrimal apparatus and nasolacrimal duct

The lacrimal gland is a serous gland situated in a shallow fossa in the superolateral aspect of the orbit (Figure 3.11). It has an orbital lobe and a smaller palpebral lobe. Twelve or more ducts release tears to moisten the conjunctiva. Excessive tears drain through the lacrimal canaliculi into the lacrimal sac situated in the lacrimal fossa, anterior to the posterior lacrimal crest. Behind the lacrimal sac, arising from the posterior lacrimal crest, is the medial palpebral ligament of the orbit. Between this and the laterally placed Whitnall's tubercle is the suspensory Lockwood's ligament which plays an important role suspending the globe in the orbit. The lacrimal sac drains inferiorly into the nasolacrimal duct, which finally opens into the inferior meatus through Hasner's valve (Figures 3.16 and 3.20).

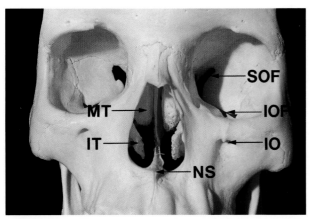

3.1

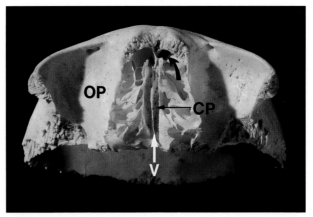

3.2

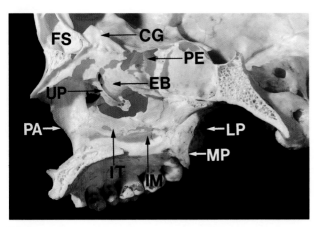

3.3

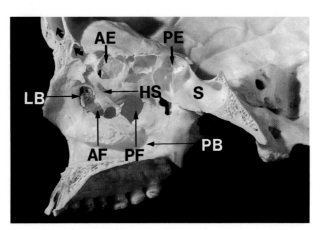

3.4

Figure **3.1**

Osteology. This anterior view of the skull demonstrates some of the bony features of the nasal cavity and orbit. The nasal spine (NS) can be seen at the base of the bony nasal septum. The prominent middle turbinate (MT) and the inferior turbinate (IT) are shown. The superior orbital fissure (SOF) and the inferior orbital fissure (IOF) are demonstrated. The inferior orbital foramen (IO) transmits the infraorbital nerve.

Figure **3.2**

Inferior aspect of the frontal bone. This inferior view shows the ethmoid notch with the depressions of the ethmoid foveolae (foveolae ethmoidales ossis frontalis) in situ. The relationship of the vomer (V) and the cribriform plate (CP) to the ethmoid foveolae, seen in Figure 3.8, is demonstrated. The curved arrow indicates the frontal recess entering the frontal sinus. The orbital plate is also shown (OP).

Figure **3.3**

Lateral wall of the nose. This half skull shows the bony features of the lateral wall of the nose. The middle turbinate and superior turbinate have been removed, opening the posterior ethmoid air cells (PE). Features demonstrated include the frontal sinus (FS), the crista galli (CG), the piriform aperture (PA), the medial (MP) and lateral (LP) pterygoid plates, the inferior turbinate (IT) and the inferior meatus (IM). The uncinate process (UP) lies anterior to the ethmoid bulla (EB). The semilunar hiatus is the two-dimensional cleft lying between these two structures.

Figure **3.4**

Lateral wall of the nose. This half skull shows the bony features of the lateral wall of the nose. The middle turbinate and superior turbinate have been removed, opening the anterior (AE) and the posterior (PE) ethmoid air cells. The small curved arrows lies within the frontal recess and the frontal sinus, respectively. Other features demonstrated include the sphenoid sinus (S), the perpendicular plate of the palatine bone (PB), the anterior (AF) and posterior (PF) fontanelles, the lacrimal bone (LB) and the semilunar hiatus (HS).

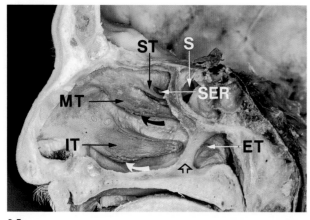

3.5

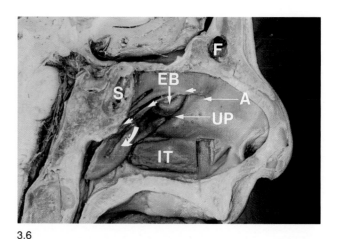

3.6

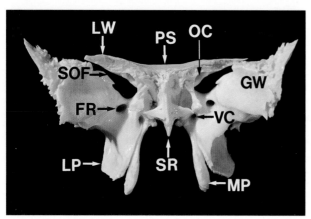

3.7

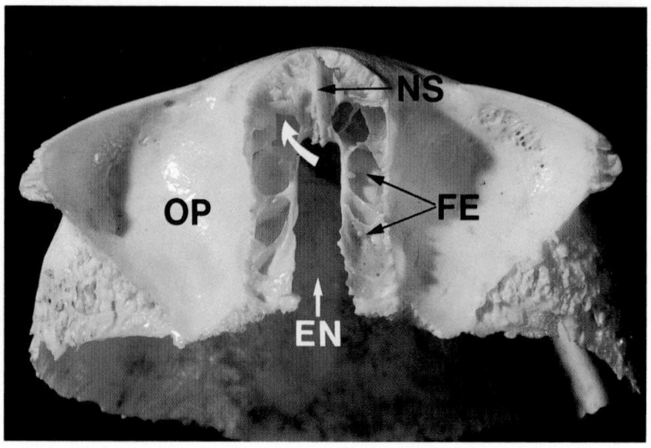

3.8

Figure **3.5**

The lateral wall of the nose. This cadaver dissection has revealed the lateral wall of the nose by removing the nasal septum. The posterior portion of the nasal septum remains at the level of the choana (open arrow). Features demonstrated include the inferior turbinate (IT), the inferior meatus (white curved arrow), the middle turbinate (MT), the middle meatus (black curved arrow), the superior turbinate (ST), the sphenoid ethmoid recess (SER) above it and the sphenoid sinus (S) and the eustachian tube orifice (ET).

Figure **3.6**

The lateral wall of the nose. This cadaver dissection has revealed more detail of the lateral wall of the nose by removing the nasal septum and reflecting the middle turbinate posteroinferiorly (curved arrow). The cut edge of the middle turbinate is emphasized with small white arrows. Other features demonstrated include the frontal sinus (F), the sphenoid sinus (S), the ethmoid bulla (EB), the uncinate process (UP) and the agger nasi (A). Part of the inferior turbinate (IT) has been resected and a fine polyethylene tube is shown protruding from the opening of the nasolacrimal duct.

Figure **3.7**

Anterior aspect of the sphenoid bone. This view demonstrates the greater (GW) and lesser wings (LW), the planum sphenoidale (PS), the superior orbital fissure (SOF), the pterygoid vidian canal (VC), the foramen rotundum (FR), the optic canal (OC), the medial (MP) and lateral (LP) pterygoid plates, and the sphenoid rostrum (SR). The lateral and the medial pterygoid plates are separated from the maxillary sinus by the pterygopalatine fossa, which receives the nerves from the foramen rotundum and the pterygoid canal.

Figure **3.8**

Inferior aspect of the frontal bone. This inferior view of a disarticulated frontal bone demonstrates the ethmoid notch (EN), which receives the crista galli and cribriform plate, the nasal spine (NS) and the ethmoid foveolae which roof the anterior and posterior ethmoid air cells (FE). The curved arrow is directed into the frontal recess and frontal sinus. The orbital plate (OP), forming the roof of the orbit is also shown.

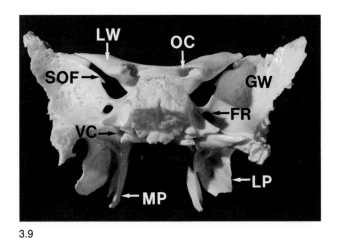

3.9

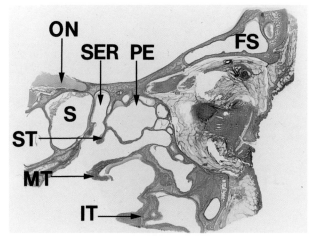

3.10

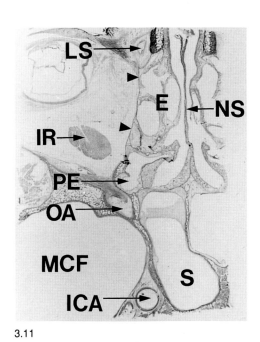

3.11

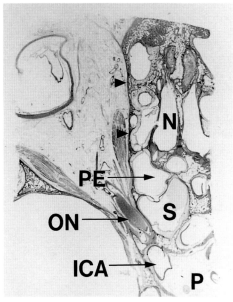

3.12

Figure **3.9**

Posterior aspect of the sphenoid bone. This view demonstrates the greater (GW) and lesser wings (LW), the pterygoid vidian canal (VC), the foramen rotundum (FR), the optic canal (OC), the medial (MP) and lateral (LP) pterygoid plates, and the superior orbital fissure (SOF).

Figure **3.10**

Parasagittal section through the orbital canal. This section demonstrates the frontal sinus (FS) extending into the orbital roof, the posterior ethmoid sinus (PE), the sphenoethmoid recess (SER), the optic nerve (ON), the superior turbinate (ST), the sphenoid sinus (S), the middle turbinate (MT) and the inferior turbinate (IT). (Masson's trichrome stain.)

Figure **3.11**

Axial section at the level of the lacrimal sac and orbital apex. This section demonstrates the lacrimal sac (LS), the anterior ethmoid air cells (E), the nasal septum (NS), the inferior rectus (IR), the lamina papyracea (arrowheads), the posterior ethmoid sinus with an Onodi's cell (PE), the orbital apex (OA), the sphenoid sinus (S), the middle cranial fossa (MCF) and the internal carotid artery (ICA). (Masson's trichrome stain.)

Figure **3.12**

Axial section at the level of the roof of the nasal cavity and the diaphragm sellae. This section demonstrates the lamina papyracea (arrowheads), the nasal cavity (N), the posterior ethmoid sinus (PE), the optic nerve (ON), the sphenoid sinus (S), the pituitary fossa (P) and the internal carotid artery (ICA). (Masson's trichrome stain.)

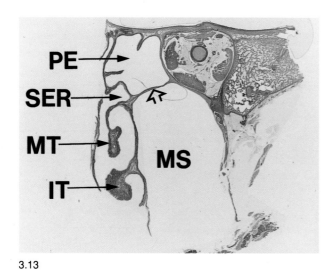

3.13

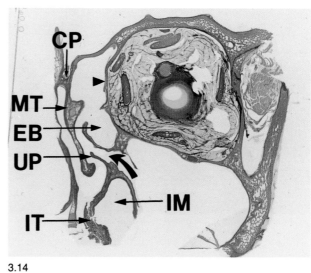

3.14

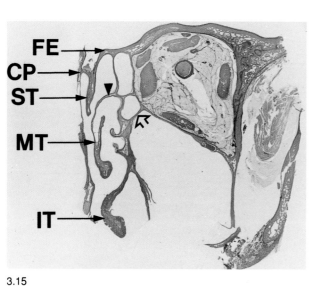

3.15

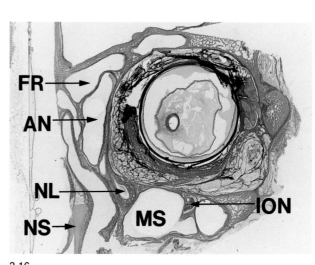

3.16

Figure **3.13**

Cross section through the posterior ethmoid sinus. The posterior ethmoid sinus (PE), the sphenoethmoid recess (SER), the middle turbinate (MT), the inferior turbinate (IT), the maxillary sinus (MS) and the ethmomaxillary plate (open arrow) are demonstrated. (Masson's trichrome stain.)

Figure **3.15**

Cross section through the posterior ethmoid sinus. The superior turbinate (ST), the middle turbinate (MT) with its horizontal insertion (arrowhead), the inferior turbinate (IT) and the ethmomaxillary plate (open arrow) are demonstrated. Note how the ethmoid fovea (FE) which roofs the ethmoid air cells lies at a much higher plane than the cribriform plate (CP). (Masson's trichrome stain.)

Figure **3.14**

Cross section through the ethmoid infundibulum and maxillary sinus ostium. The cribriform plate (CP), the lamina papyracea (arrowhead), the middle turbinate (MT), the ethmoid bulla (EB), the uncinate process (UP), the inferior turbinate (IT) and the inferior meatus (IM) are demonstrated. The curved arrow passes through the maxillary sinus ostium into the ethmoid infundibulum. (Masson's trichrome stain.)

Figure **3.16**

Coronal section through the anterior ethmoid. This section demonstrates the frontal recess (FR), the agger nasi (AN), the nasolacrimal duct (NL), the nasal septum (NS), the maxillary sinus (MS) and the infraorbital nerve (ION). (Masson's trichrome stain.)

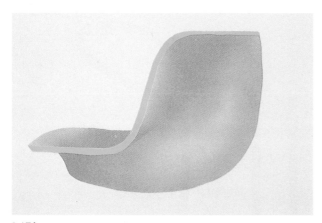

3.17A

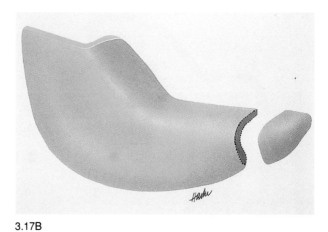

3.17B

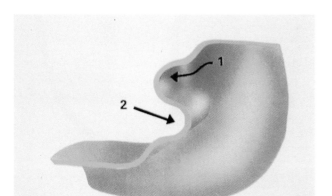

3.18

Figure **3.17**

The middle turbinate. These diagrams show the ground lamella of the middle turbinate from laterally (A) and medially (B). The posterior tip of the lateral view has been divided to demonstrate the vertical and horizontal plates of the turbinate.

Figure **3.18**

The lateral sinus. This diagram of the middle turbinate demonstrates how the ground lamella may be distorted by the lateral sinus (arrow 1) and the posterior ethmoid (arrow 2).

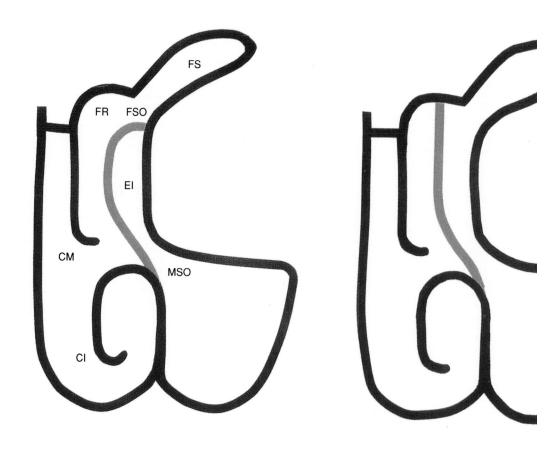

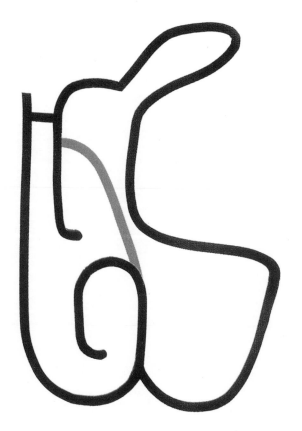

Figure **3.19**

The insertion of the uncinate process. These diagrams simplify the variations of the insertion of the uncinate process and its effect upon the drainage pattern of the frontal recess. EI, ethmoid infundibulum; FR, frontal recess, FSO, frontal sinus ostium; FS, frontal sinus; MSO, maxillary sinus ostium; CM, concha media; CI, concha inferior.

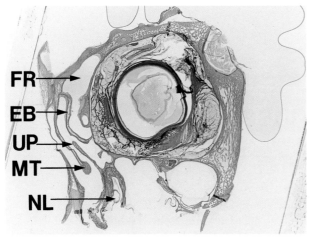

3.20

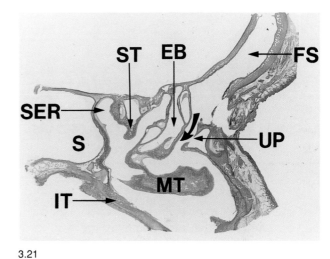

3.21

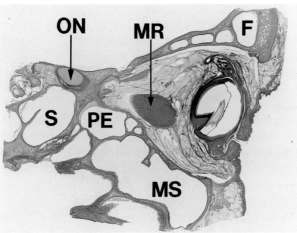

3.22

Figure **3.20**

Cross section through the ethmoid infundibulum anterior to the maxillary sinus ostium. This coronal section demonstrates the frontal recess (FR), the ethmoid bulla (EB), the uncinate process (UP), the middle turbinate (MT) and the nasolacrimal duct (NL). (Masson's trichrome stain.)

Figure **3.22**

Parasagittal section through the sphenoid sinus. This section demonstrates the frontal sinus (F), the medial rectus (MR), the optic nerve (ON), the sphenoid sinus (S), the posterior ethmoid sinus (PE) and the maxillary sinus (MS). (Masson's trichrome stain.)

Figure **3.21**

Parasagittal section through the cribriform plate. This section demonstrates the frontal sinus (FS), the uncinate process (UP), the ethmoid bulla (EB), the superior turbinate (ST), the sphenoethmoid recess (SER), the sphenoid sinus (S), the inferior turbinate (IT), and the middle turbinate (MT). The curved arrow shows the path from the frontal recess into the ethmoid infundibulum. (Masson's trichrome stain).

4

Basic principles of radiography of the nasal cavity and paranasal sinuses

For many years rhinologists and radiologists have had to rely upon plain radiographs of the paranasal sinuses for assistance in the diagnosis and management of paranasal sinus disease. The information gleaned from these films is mainly relevant to the general condition of the larger paranasal sinuses (especially the frontal, maxillary and sphenoid sinuses), and yields minimal information about the delicate bony anatomic or mucosal changes that may be present in the ethmoid air cells of the lateral wall of the nose. With the development of functional endoscopic sinus surgery, such imaging has proved inadequate.

Conventional or plain radiographs usually involve four projections; Caldwell's projection, the lateral projection, Water's projection and the submento-vertical projection. While these films are adequate for a basic or preliminary assessment of the larger paranasal sinuses they fail to demonstrate adequately the anterior ethmoid sinuses, the upper nasal cavities, the surrounding soft tissue or the frontal recesses clearly. Nevertheless, plain radiographs continue to have a place in the diagnosis and management of acute sinusitis and will readily demonstrate the presence of an air–fluid interface or a totally opacified sinus (Figures 4.1 and 4.2). A repeat Water's view is generally appropriate for following the clinical progress of acute maxillary or frontal sinus infections.

POLYTOMOGRAPHY

Conventional tomography, especially hypocycloidal polytomography can provide excellent images of the bony margins of the sinuses and thin bony leaflets in the ethmoid labyrinth. The development of these imaging techniques was fundamental in the evolution of functional endoscopic sinus surgery. Conventional tomography has now been superseded by computed tomography (CT). Conventional tomography still maintains some advantages: in the ready availability of the equipment required to take conventional tomograms, and in its ability to record images in the sagittal plane while the patient remains in a comfortable position, unlike direct sagittal plane CTs, which require the patient to assume awkward and uncomfortable positions. The major disadvantage of conventional tomography is the dose of radiation administered, which is significantly greater than that delivered during CT. This is a particular disadvantage with respect to the lens of the eye. The quality of conventional tomograms is further diminished by the appearance of phantom artifacts which may obscure small anatomic structures and limited areas of significant disease. The soft-tissue resolution with CT is far superior to that with conventional tomography.

CT is currently regarded as the imaging modality of choice for the paranasal sinuses. It should be used to complement noninvasive diagnostic endoscopy in the assessment of the individual patient, and it will help to demonstrate normal and pathologic anatomy prior to commencing surgery.

There are many advantages to be gained from using CT as opposed to conventional tomography. The contrast and resolution are of higher quality with CT. This helps to differentiate minor opacities that may be obscured by the blurring effect of the conventional tomogram, and bony decalcifications that may be concealed by inflammatory changes. In a similar manner, malignant bony infiltration can be more readily differentiated from inflammatory changes.

COMPUTED TOMOGRAPHY

In CT, a well-collimated slit-like beam is produced from the X-ray tube. This tube-detector unit, housed in the gantry encircles the patient being examined, moving in 1° intervals while X-rays are continuously produced. These projected rays pass through the patient, some being absorbed, others passing through unchanged. An array of detectors receives the X-ray signals which have been attenuated during the passage through the various tissues. The quality of the image depends primarily upon the number of picture elements (pixels) used, which will either be on a 256×256 or a 512×512 matrix. With the knowledge of the scan thickness, the volume of the picture elements can be measured and stored as units named voxels. The absorption of X-ray photons in a voxel is related to the average absorption coefficient. The image produced is a reflection of the number of photons absorbed by each voxel. This density distribution is readily detected electronically, leading to production of a superior image.

CT has a tremendous capacity for density resolution, and 4000 grades of density, from air to metal, can be identified, which allows the differentiation of all clinically relevant tissue. These density grades are measured in Hounsfield units (HU) and range from −1000 to +3000 HU. These different densities are projected as different tones of gray on an electronic screen. Unfortunately, the human eye is only capable of differentiating approximately 40 different tones of the same color. To overcome this, the computer is able to manipulate the electronic raw data within variable electronic 'windows'. Within a given window, the density values will be shown as different shades of gray while, outside that particular window, the greater density values will be shown as white and the lesser densities as black. This has the advantage that the raw data can be manipulated by the computer to provide information about both bony structures (using a wide window setting), and soft-tissue structures (using a narrow window setting), from only one exposure to the X-rays (the raw data). Each window is centered at a specific value. This determines which density of tissue will be displayed with the medium tone of gray. The recommended window width and the window centers vary with each anatomic region. For imaging of the paranasal sinuses and the ostiomeatal complex, a wide window setting (between 2000 and 3000 HU) is used, centered around −250 HU. This usually demonstrates both the bone and the soft tissues adequately. When soft-tissue pathology is to be emphasized, the scanner is set with a narrower window width of 300 centered around +65 HU.

Other parameters are also of importance including the dose, milliamperes/per second (MAS), kilovoltage (kVP) and the slice thickness. There is a linear relationship between dose and MAS, with the dose increasing as the MAS increases. The dosage to the patient is also dependent upon the voltage, filters and collimators used, as well as the slice thickness. The MAS setting will vary depending on the noise level, kVP, patient size and the scan slice thickness. For imaging the paranasal sinuses, the kVP is usually set at 125 and the MAS at 450.

Resolution

High-resolution computed tomography (HRCT) involves the scanning of thin sections for the enhancement of bony details. High-resolution scanning is made possible by the use of special reconstruction software available with most CT scanners.

The best high-resolution images are achieved with the thinnest slices. This improved spatial resolution enables one to see bony microanatomy, subtle erosions and fractures. Some of the volume elements (voxels), will contain both bone and soft tissue and the gray value displayed in the image is based on the average absorption value for that voxel. It is therefore inaccurate for the separate tissue types. If there is a large difference between the tissue densities within a voxel, streak artifacts will appear on the image (Figure 4.3). This is also known as the partial volume effect. This artifact may be diminished by reducing the scan thickness.

Imaging of the paranasal sinuses is usually conducted with a 4–5 mm scan thickness with the table moving in 3–4 mm increments. This allows some overlap of contiguous scans to facilitate reformatting in a different plane or three-dimensional reconstruction. The scan time, for each slice, is usually between 5 and 7 s.

The raw data of regions with a large difference in contrast, i.e. bone soft-tissue edges, may be reconstructed directly or subsequently into high-resolution images by special algorithms that improve spatial resolution. This creates more clearly defined images of regions such as the inner ear and the paranasal sinuses, but it is an inappropriate technique for the imaging of soft-tissue regions. The image is more likely to be distorted by noise and artifact with this technique; however, this may be reduced by using a wide window and a thin scan slice. Wide windows are unable to differentiate small variations in density. In contrast, the narrow window enables separation of very small density differences at the expense of bony detail.

Artifacts

The image produced with CT can be degraded by artifacts of various origin and these may obscure the differentiation of contiguous soft tissue or soft tissue and tumor. A grainy appearance on the image is due to noise. This is caused by slight variations of the density value measured by the scanner for substances of a fixed density. This effect may be limited by increasing the MAS or the scan thickness in areas of soft tissue, but it has little effect in areas of high density contrast. Ring artifacts may be caused when individual detector channels show slight differences in signal output. This may result from infrequent unit calibration and may be corrected by a balancing algorithm. Streak artifacts, as already mentioned, appear if there are sudden changes in tissue density within a voxel. These may be limited by an extended balancing algorithm used while at the raw data stage or by reducing the scan slice thickness. Careful patient positioning and gantry angulation may allow such areas of density change (e.g. dental fillings) to be avoided.

X-ray tubes produce radiation of varying levels, the lower levels being attenuated to a greater degree and thereby increasing the spectrum of energy levels measured. This effect is known as beam hardening. Much of this effect may be reduced by beam filtering and the addition of a correcting algorithm before scanning the patient. The artifacts produced are most pronounced in areas where high-density structures are in close proximity to low-density structures. Careful positioning of the patient, and careful filtering of the beam before entry into the patient, may lead to a reduction in such artifacts. Artifacts due to dental amalgam may be avoided by scanning in a different plane. Some artifacts may be caused by movement of the patient. This may be reduced by explaining to the patient what events to expect during the examination and by ensuring that they are comfortably positioned and well supported. The patient should be asked to refrain from swallowing and breathing at the start of the scan time.

Table 4.1 The scanning plane that will afford the most information about an individual structure.

Structure	Axial	Coronal
Maxillary sinus		
anterior wall	•	
posterior wall	•	
medial wall		•
roof/orbital floor		•
Frontal sinus		
anterior wall	•	
posterior wall	•	
floor		•
Sphenoid sinus		
anterior	•	
posterior	•	
lateral		•
floor		•
Ethmoid sinus		
lateral wall	•	•
roof		•
Ostiomeatal complex		•
Pterygopalatine fossa	•	
Superior orbital fissure		•
Optic nerve	•	•a
Cribriform plate		•
Turbinates		•

aParasagittal scans of this region provide particularly good visualization of the canal of the optic nerve.

Enlargement

Specific areas of interest may be enlarged by one or two methods. The first, magnification, involves the expansion of each picture element. With this technique there is no increase in detail and the tissue interfaces may become stepped. With the second technique, zooming, a segment of the image is coned to produce increased detail resolution. The zoom factors vary from 1 to 10, the larger zoom

Table **4.2** The ideal scanning plane for a number of conditions.

Disorder	Axial	Coronal	Sagittal	3D CT
Trauma	•	•	•	•
Benign polyposis		•		
Inflammatory disease		•		
Malignancy	•	•	•	•
Mucocele/pyocele	•	•	±	±
Congenital anomalies	•	•		•

factor being associated with smaller pixels and therefore greater definition. The latter technique is more appropriate when studying the paranasal sinuses, and zoom factors between 4 and 6 are generally applied.

Projections

Coronal scans of the paranasal sinuses are preferred to axial scans because they allow more appropriate orientation of the anatomy and pathology in the perspective by which they will be approached by the endoscopist. This orientation also allows more accurate visualization of those structures that lie parallel to the infraorbital line, such as the orbital roof and floor, the roof of the nasal cavity, the ethmoid and the sphenoid sinus. This is of particular value when it is suspected that disease or fracture have penetrated these structures.

A cooperative patient with good neck extension is essential for adequate scanning in the coronal axial plane. Many elderly patients may not be able to comply with this; in this event, the problem can be overcome by the computer's ability to reconstruct images in a different plane to that studied from the information within the data store. This overcomes some of the problems encountered with patients having limited neck extension or scanners with limited gantry angulation. In these circumstances, it may be preferable to scan the patient in the axial plane and reconstruct the images in the coronal plane (Figure 4.4). This ability to reconstruct the images enables the radiologist to study any abnormality in a variety of planes, including the sagittal plane. Unfortunately reconstruction diminishes the definition of the scan and may obscure minor mucosal or bony defects.

For scanning in the coronal plane, the patient is positioned either prone or supine and the gantry is angled to lie perpendicular to the infraorbitomeatal line (also known as Reid's line). In the supine position, the neck is hyperextended at the gantry end of the table, and if the patient is prone, then the chin is fixed and supported after extending the neck. Initially a lateral 'scout' scan is taken, and if necessary the gantry angulation is modified to take into account special problems as limited extension of the neck or metal dental fillings that may degrade the image (Figure 4.5). The patient is then scanned from the posterior margin of the sphenoid sinus to the frontal sinus.

The technique used for axial scanning is not dissimilar to that used for coronal scanning. The patient is usually positioned supine with the gantry parallel to the orbitomeatal line. The limits of the scan extend from the alveolar ridge to the top of the frontal sinus. For both planes, the scan thickness is

4–5 mm and the table moves in 3–4 mm increments (Figure 4.6).

Imaging of the paranasal sinuses in the axial and coronal planes each have their own separate advantages and disadvantages, as illustrated in Tables 4.1 and 4.2. Axial scans are generally regarded as being excellent for the evaluation of the anterior and posterior walls of the paranasal sinuses and the pterygopalatine fossa, and especially the relationships of the optic nerve to the posterior ethmoid and sphenoid sinuses. Coronal scans more clearly demonstrate abnormalities of the paranasal sinuses, especially those involving the lateral wall of the nose, as well as the nasopharyngeal and parapharyngeal regions. Multiplanar scanning is considered the ideal; however, time, patient compliance and the increased radiation dose restrict the use of this more extensive examination when benign disease is being investigated.

Administration of contrast

Intravenous contrast is not used routinely during the investigation of benign inflammatory disease and is administered at the discretion of the radiologist. Ideally, contrast should be administered with an automatic injector. Approximately 80–100 ml of nonionic contrast is given at the rate of 1 ml/s and a rapid sequential series is taken. Abnormalities will enhance if there is increased vascularity and the degree of enhancement can be estimated by comparison with the enhancement of the great vessels. Contrast is indicated if vascular abnormalities or malignancy are suspected from either the history or diagnostic examination. The vascularity of the lesion as well as its relationship to the major vessels can be assessed preoperatively. If embolization is being contemplated, angiography may be used to complement the CT findings. Narrow window settings delineate the extent of soft tissue and loss of the fat planes may indicate malignancy, whereas a wide window setting will help to demonstrate the bony features, especially erosion due to benign or malignant lesions.

The administration of contrast may help to distinguish between active and chronic inflammatory disease as mucosal enhancement is visible in cases of active inflammation. Intravenous contrast is certainly indicated when inflammatory sinus disease is complicated by abscess formation, thrombosis, intracranial or intraorbital spread of infection. The distinction between allergic and inflammatory polyps may also be aided by contrast administration as inflammatory polyps have been noted to enhance whereas allergic polyps do not.

The administration of intravenous contrast does have some disadvantages. The major medical disadvantage is the occurrence of a potentially fatal anaphylactic reaction to the contrast agent. The major nonmedical disadvantage is the expense of nonionic intravenous contrast. In general intravenous contrast enhancement is limited to those cases of tumors, vascular lesions and complicated paranasal disease. It is rarely administered in cases of uncomplicated inflammatory and allergic sinus disease because of its cost.

Interpretation and reporting

The system developed to interpret and report the images will depend on the individual radiologist's preferences. With such complex anatomy, and any pathological abnormality further distorting this anatomy, it is wise to develop a systematic approach and thereby avoid omitting important details. A reporting scheme has been developed by the authors which not only allows thorough and accurate examination of the radiological images, but is also of value in standardizing reports, and in allowing data collected over a period of time or from different pathologies to be reviewed with ease (Table 4.3).

Comparison of Computed Tomography with Magnetic Resonance Imaging

Magnetic resonance (MR) imaging involves rapidly changing magnetic fields instead of ionizing radiation. MR depends upon the physical and the biochemical properties of the tissue, i.e. the hydrogen density, and the T1 and T2 (the longitudinal and the transverse magnetic) relaxation constants. The other important parameters that influence MR imaging are the pulse repetition time (TR time) and the echo delay (TE). A pulse sequence with a short TR and a short TE is called a T1-weighted sequence. A sequence with a long TR and a long TE is called a T2-weighted sequence. Fat and marrow produce a high signal intensity (a brighter

Table 4.3 Sinus CT reporting scheme.

	Sinuses	Drainage pathways	Lateral wall	Septum and bony walls
Regions examined	1 frontal 2 maxillary 3 anterior ethmoid 4 posterior ethmoid 5 sphenoid	6 frontal recess 7 ostium 8 infundibulum 9 superior meatus 10 sphenoethmoid recess	11 aggar nasi 12 uncinate process 13 Haller's cell 14 middle turbinate 15 ethmoid bulla 16 inferior turbinate 17 lateral recess	18 nasal septum 19 lamina papyracea
Structural variation	hypoplasia [1,2,5] septated [2] accessory ostium [2] pneumatized roof [2] Caldwell–Luc procedure [2] antrostromy [2]	patent compromised occluded	absent [12,14,15,16] large [all] large+compromise [all] large+disease [all] pneumatized [12,14,16] pneumatized+disease [12,14,16] paradoxiacal deviation [14] previous excision [all] medially bent [12]	deviation/spur [18] narrowing ostiomeatal complex [18] perforation [18] pneumatized [18] eroded lamina papyracea [19]
Pathology seen	mucus/pus minimal mucosal thickening severe mucosal thickening polypoidal single cyst/polyp opacity mucocele antrochoanal polyp air–fluid level fungal mass reactive osteitis erosion septae		osteoma soft-tissue tumor foreign body rhinolith	

* Numbers in brackets indicate the structures affected.

image), water and inflammation produce a low signal intensity (a darker image), whereas bone and air produce no signal. The physics of MR will be discussed later in more detail.

CT and MR imaging have added a third dimension to radiologic imaging of the paranasal sinuses. It is now possible to detect early disease, be it inflammatory or neoplastic, and the spread of such disease, either intracranially or into the orbit, is well demonstrated by both modalities. MR imaging is complementary to CT because of its superior soft tissue resolution, and each modality has independent benefits.

The particular advantages of CT over MR imaging include the following.

i *Bony detail*: CT identifies bony details such as the proximity of the orbital floor to the site of a middle meatal antrostomy, the extent of pneumatization of the ethmoid air cells, the location of the natural maxillary sinus ostium, septations of the sphenoid sinus and the position of the internal carotid artery, as well as the degree of pneumatization and depth of the frontal sinus.

ii *Cost*: at present CT is significantly less expensive and more readily available than MR imaging.

iii *Examination time*: CT takes only seconds per scan slice, whereas MR imaging at present requires several minutes per slice. This increases the likelihood of patient movement and therefore degradation of the scan.

iv *Patient comfort*: MR scanners tend to be noisier and more confining than CT scanners, and therefore patients with claustrophobia may not be able to tolerate the procedure.

The main advantages of MR imaging over CT include the following:

i *Superior soft-tissue discrimination*: this permits better assessment of the interface between a pathologic mass and the surrounding normal structures, and rarely requires the administration of intravenous contrast.

ii *Multiplanar capability*: any anatomic plane may be examined without the patient being asked to take up an uncomfortable position and without the application of low-resolution computer reformations. The coronal plane is usually the most informative plane when examining the head and neck.

iii *Vascular anatomy*: vascular structures are readily seen without intravenous contrast and are easily separated from other soft-tissue structures. MR angiograms may soon supersede conventional angiograms.

iv *Artifacts*: on MR, the artifacts from dental amalgam and cortical bone are insignificant in contrast to those on CT, in which significant image degradation can occur.

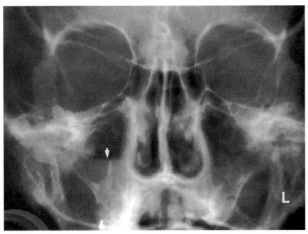

4.1

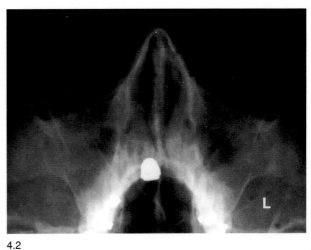

4.2

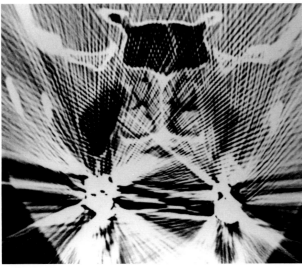

4.3

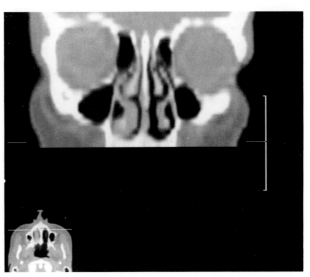

4.4

Figure **4.1**

Acute maxillary sinusitis. This plain radiograph clearly demonstrates an air–fluid level in the right maxillary sinus (arrow). There is also some mucosal thickening in the left maxillary antrum. Patients should not undergo CT during the acute phase of an uncomplicated sinus infection, as the acute inflammatory swelling prevents the ostiomeatal complex from being clearly visualized. The maximum information is gleaned from scans conducted when the patient is in a quiescent phase.

Figure **4.3**

Dental amalgam causing streak artifacts. This CT scan shows the extensive artifacts that can occur from metallic dental amalgam. This phenomenon is also known as the partial volume effect.

Figure **4.2**

Chronic maxillary sinusitis. The limitations of plain radiographs are demonstrated by this Water's view. There is diffuse mucosal thickening in both maxillary sinuses which is typical of chronic maxillary sinusitis. Little information can be gained from plain radiographs about the ostiomeatal complex or the adjacent ethmoid sinuses in patients with recurrent or persistent sinusitis.

Figure **4.4**

Coronal reconstruction. This coronal reconstruction from axial CT scans demonstrates the ostiomeatal complex. Unfortunately, the anatomic definition is not as clear as that seen in direct coronal scans. Coronal reconstruction is usually limited to those patients who are unable to cooperate with direct scanning, because of limited neck movement.

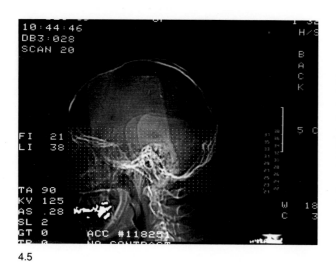

4.5

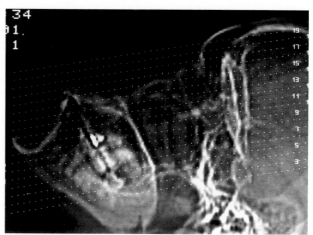

4.6

Figure **4.5**

The lateral topogram (the tope or scout image). This topogram shows the scan lines for CT of the paranasal sinuses in the axial plane. The scanning lines lie parallel to the infraorbitomeatal line.

Figure **4.6**

For coronal scans, the topogram will demonstrate the scanning lines perpendicular to the infraorbitomeatal line. The gantry angulation may be altered to avoid metal dental fillings which will degrade the image.

5

The role of conventional sinus radiographs in paranasal sinus disease

Martyn Mendelsohn   Arnold Noyek

For many decades, plain sinus radiographs provided the family practitioner and the otolaryngologist with a road map of sinus pathology. The antrum, which was formerly the putative focus of sinus disease, is well displayed by plain radiographs. However modern theory focuses upon the importance of the ethmoids in sinus infection. This shift in emphasis dramatically increased the role of computed tomography (CT) scans, which can image the ethmoids and provide a guide to endoscopic surgery. In this light, modern reviews have underemphasized the role of plain radiography. Has the pendulum swung too far? This chapter discusses the role of plain sinus films in the current era, and indicates the range of pathology which can be imaged by plain sinus radiography.

TECHNIQUE

The standard views include the Water's (occipitomental), Caldwell (occipitofrontal), lateral and basal (submentovertical) views. Many supplementary films are available, including the panoramic tomogram and orbital oblique views. The features displayed on each are summarized in Table 5.1. Technical data is covered in greater detail by Valvasori et al (1982).

Table 5.1 Principal features displayed in each view

Water's view
    maxillary antrum
    anterior and middle ethmoid cells
    orbital floor

Caldwell's view
    posterior ethmoid cells
    frontal sinuses
    template for osteoplastic flap

Lateral view
    sphenoid
    antrum, frontal sinuses

Basal view
    sphenoid

Panoramic tomogram
    antral floor
    dental roots

Water's view

The Water's view is the primary view to observe the maxillary antra and the anterior ethmoid sinuses. The orbits, nasal cavities and zygomatic arches are also well seen.

Caldwell view

This view highlights frontoethmoidal disease and the orbits. In this view, the patient's face is in contact with the film holder. This ensures minimal magnification of the frontal bone so that the image can be the basis for a frontal sinus template in osteoplastic flap surgery.

Lateral view

This is the only view that can consistently display an air–fluid level in the sphenoid sinus. The transparency of the sinuses is difficult to judge due to the overlap of the two sides. The sella turcica and nasopharynx are well seen.

Basal view

This view provides comparison of each sphenoid sinus, and also the ethmoid sinuses and nasal cavities. The mastoid air cells may be included in this view in patients who have associated ear symptoms.

Panoramic tomogram (Panorex, Orthopantomogram)

Although not a standard paranasal sinus view, the panoramic tomogram can provide unique information on the floor of the antrum, the pterygopalatine surface of the sinuses and the teeth. This view is invaluable to investigate any case of dental involvement. Panoramic machines are now commonly available in the dental department of most hospitals.

RADIOLOGIC FEATURES

Interpretation of plain radiographs requires an assessment of bone, soft tissue and air. Radiologic signs are summarized in Tables 5.2 and 5.3. These signs must always be correlated with the clinical picture.

Table **5.2** Radiologic signs in paranasal sinus disease (from Zizmor and Noyek, 1976).

Decreased aeration and luminal opacification

Mucosal thickening

Cyst formation

Soft-tissue mass

Air–fluid level

Emphysema

Calcification

Ossification

One or more adult or embryonic teeth

Foreign body (bodies)

Alterations in bony walls

Table **5.3** Alterations in bony walls.

Decalcification

Osteolysis

Dehiscence

Fracture(s)

Osteoblastosis or hyperostosis

Expansion and displacement of bony walls

Decreased luminal volume

Sequestrum (sequestra)

Anatomy

The role of each view in imaging the sinuses is summarized in Table 5.I. The plain films indicate the size and symmetry between the two sides. The frontal sinuses are frequently asymmetric and may be absent. The thickness and integrity of the bony walls are well seen. Anatomic variations, such as hypoplasia, bony sclerosis and the presence of a sinus septum, are a useful guide for surgeons undertaking antral surgery or frontal sinus trephine.

The panoramic tomogram demonstrates the maxillary teeth and the antral floor. The relationship of the tooth roots has some variability, but generally the two premolars and the first two molar teeth have roots in the floor of the maxillary sinus. Tooth roots, supernumary teeth and unerupted teeth seen on plain films may be associated with cysts and antral pathology.

Paranasal sinus disease

Radiologic abnormalities have been demonstrated in 40% of asymptomatic patients on CT (Yanagisa and Smith, 1976). Most abnormalities are mucosal thickening or polyps in the ethmoid sinus and the floor of the antra. This reinforces the importance of correlating the radiologic signs with the clinical features.

Acute maxillary, frontal and sphenoid sinusitis can be identified by mucosal thickening and the presence of fluid. Fluid is most reliably indicated by an air fluid level. Whether the fluid is pus, serous transudate, blood, cerebrospinal fluid or other must be established on clinical grounds. Generalized mucosal thickening without fluid may indicate acute or chronic inflammatory change. Total luminal opacification may be the result of empyema or a soft-tissue mass, or may reflect thicker bone or soft tissue overlying that sinus. In cases suggesting luminal opacification, an alternate view is mandatory to verify the presence of pathology.

Chronic sinusitis, resulting from infection or allergy, may be evidenced by localized or diffuse soft-tissue thickening or cysts. Osteitis is suggested by bony sclerosis or rarefaction. Polypoid disease may obliterate an entire sinus. An antrochoanal polyp may be seen in the lateral view. Antral cysts warrant a panoramic view, to establish the relationship between the cyst and any normal or abnormal teeth.

Unlike the other paranasal sinuses, ethmoid pathology is usually identified on plain radiographs by obliteration of multiple small cells rather than mucosal thickening or fluid level changes within a sinus. Consequently, in comparison with CT scans, plain radiographs have limited resolution and hence ability in identifying early ethmoid changes. The newly recognized importance of ethmoid sinusitis and the increasing vogue for functional endoscopic sinus surgery have resulted in the increased popularity of CT scanning in imaging of the ethmoid region in chronic sinusitis.

Other radiologic signs, which are listed in Table 5.2 and 5.3, may result from complications of sinus infection, benign or malignant tumor, trauma or other disorder. These often require further investigation, as indicated by the clinical presentation.

THE ROLE OF PLAIN RADIOGRAPHS

Sinusitis is the most common health care complaint in the USA, affecting more than 31 million people (Havas et al 1988). As a community problem, most cases of sinusitis are diagnosed by the family practitioner, based upon the history and physical examination. In many cases, the patient responds to medical management and no imaging is necessary.

There are many situations in which plain radiography may be used as a screening examination to diagnose paranasal sinus pathology (Table 5.4). The symptoms may be atypical. The clinician may be reluctant to prescribe antibiotics, or the patient reluctant to take antibiotics, until the diagnosis is more

---

Table 5.4 Indications for plain radiography.

Screening

   sinusitis

   trauma

   foreign body

   suspected complications

Preoperative

   antral puncture, intranasal antrostomy,

   radical antrostomy

   frontal sinus trephine

   osteoplastic flap template (Caldwell's view)

Assessment of dental disease

definite. The symptoms may persist despite an initial course of antibiotics. Plain radiographs may be useful in screening for some complications of sinus disease, such as mucocele, orbital abscess, osteomyelitis, Pott's puffy tumor, etc. However, definitive management of these complications invariably requires CT examinations.

Plain radiographs are ideally suited to screen for a widespread community illness such as sinusitis. Most acute infections involve more than one sinus and are well displayed on plain radiographs. Plain radiography is cheaper and more readily available than CT or magnetic resonance imaging. Sinus radiographs can often be obtained on the day on which radiography is performed, for immediate review by the referring practitioner. The reduction in cost for imaging such a large-scale problem results in a major health savings compared to other investigations, which are substantially more expensive. If plain sinus radiographs appear normal despite strong clinical suspicion, the clinician may then choose to proceed to more elaborate and expensive tests based upon clinical features. Furthermore, the clinician may recognize one or more sinister radiographic signs that also indicate the need for further investigation.

Dental disease is a well-recognized cause of sinusitis that may be resistant to simple therapy. Plain sinus radiographs supplemented by panoramic and dental views display the antrum and coexistent dental pathology, including apical disease, abnormal or supernumary teeth, dental cysts and the presence of an oroantral fistula.

Not all patients with sinusitis want or need endoscopic sinus surgery. Plain radiographs provide the surgeon with a 'road map' before antral puncture, intranasal antrostomy, radical antrostomy and frontal sinus trephine. The radiographs can reveal the presence of a hypoplastic sinus, bony septae or thickened bony walls, and so improve the safety and efficiency of the surgical procedure. The Caldwell view provides the template for osteoplastic frontal sinus surgery.

Plain radiographs may aid the localization or identification of foreign bodies. The exact position can be correlated by observing multiple views. Plain films are useful in screening for facial trauma, although clear evidence of complex maxillofacial trauma requires CT scanning.

Figures 5.1–5.8 illustrate some of the potentials and pitfalls of plain radiographs of the paranasal sinuses. In Figures 5.1–5.4 are shown cases in which the plain radiographs provide adequate information for clinical decision making. The subsequent Figures illustrate cases that required CT evaluation.

CONCLUSION

Despite the current excitement surrounding CT of the paranasal sinuses, plain radiographs still have several clinical applications. The discerning clinician selects the most cost-efficient and time-efficient test that can provide adequate information.

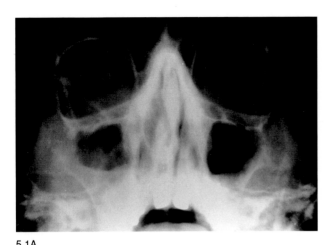

5.1A

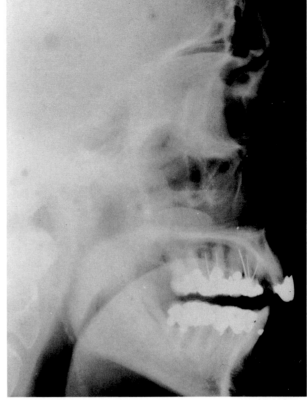

5.1B

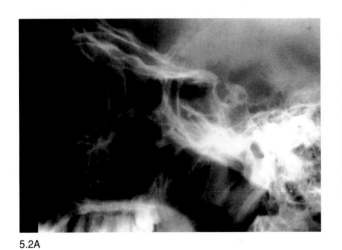

5.2A

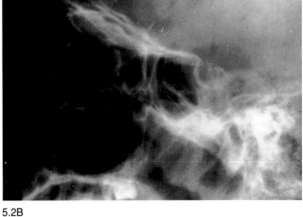

5.2B

Figure **5.1**

Plain radiography. (A) The material in the lower half of the left antrum (on the upright Water's view) has a concave meniscus, diagnostic of an air–fluid level. The density in the right maxillary sinus has a convex surface, characteristic of a mucous retention cyst in the floor of the antrum. The comparison is striking. (B) The superimposed images of the fluid level and the cyst are well seen in the lateral view.

Figure **5.2**

Sphenoidal sinusitis. The sphenoidal fluid level seen on plain radiographs (A) resolved with conservative treatment (B).

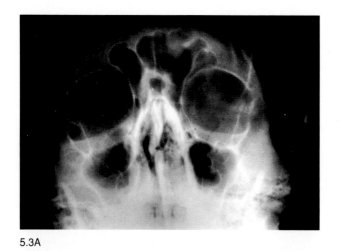

5.3A

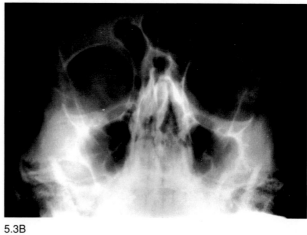

5.3B

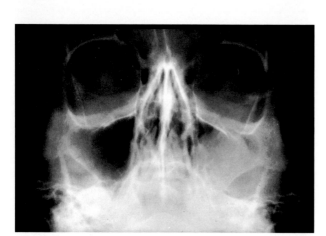

5.4

Figure **5.3**

Barotrauma and hematoma. This patient experienced left frontal pain upon descent in an aeroplane. (A) The plain radiograph demonstrates a soft-tissue mass in the superior left frontal sinus. (B) A similar film 2 weeks later shows resolution, confirming the diagnosis of frontal sinus hematoma secondary to barotrauma.

Figure **5.4**

Left antral mucous retention or serous cyst. The superior surface of the lesion is smooth and convex, and there is a pocket of air in the antrum. The plain radiograph is adequate for the diagnosis of a large mucous retention cyst arising from the lower portion of the antrum.

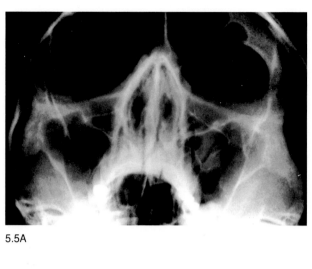

5.5A

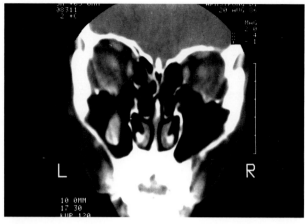

5.5B

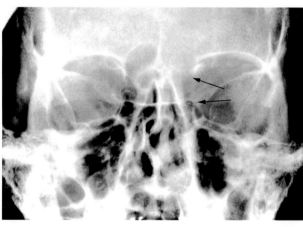

5.6A

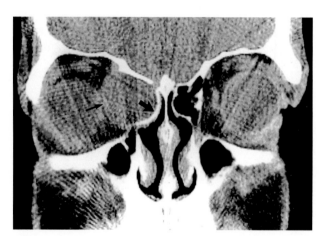

5.6B

Figure **5.5**

Antral roof polyp. (A) Plain radiography (Water's view) demonstrated an unusual finding in the left antrum. This required CT evaluation (B) which revealed a polyp hanging from the antral roof on a long stalk.

Figure **5.6**

(A) The plain radiograph demonstrates a left ethmoid opacity with bone destruction of the lamina papyracea (arrows). (B) CT was required to display the full extent of the soft-tissue expansion into the orbit by an ethmoid mucocele (small arrow). The thick arrow indicates displaced thickened bone.

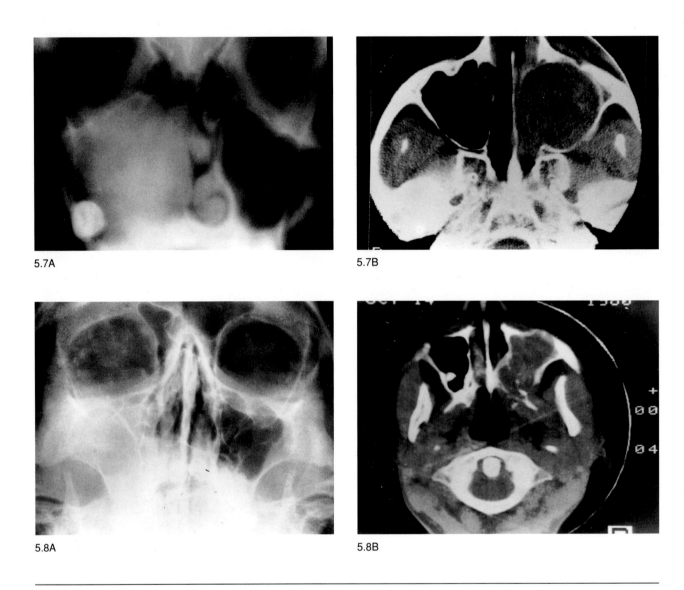

5.7A

5.7B

5.8A

5.8B

Figure **5.7**

Dentigerous cyst. (A) The antrum appears opaque and
expanded, and the crown of an ectopic tooth is clearly
displayed on complex motion tomography. (B) The axial CT
demonstrates that the mass is cystic, extrinsic in origin and has
expanded to virtually replace the antrum and adjacent nasal
cavity.

Figure **5.8**

Completely opaque left antrum without bone destruction. The
patient had a 15-year history of 'chronic sinusitis'. (A) On the
plain radiograph complete antral opacification gives no clue as
to the nature of the antral pathology. No bone destruction is
seen. (B) CT demonstrates a solid mass eroding the posterior
antral wall and destroying the pterygoid plates. Biopsy revealed
malignant schwannoma.

6

The normal anatomy of the paranasal sinuses as seen with Computed Tomography and Magnetic Resonance Imaging

The radiologist must be familiar with the anatomy of the ethmoid labyrinth, the larger paranasal sinuses and their associated ventilation and drainage channels in the lateral nasal wall. The relevant anatomy is described in this chapter in the axial, sagittal and coronal planes, with additional information about the more commonly occurring anatomic variants. Each radiologist will need to develop their own scheme for the systematic reporting of computed tomographs of this challenging anatomic area.

THE EXTERNAL NOSE

The external nose is the first structure visualized in the coronal scans (Figure 6.1). If the frontal sinuses are prominent, they will also appear in the most anterior scans.

THE FRONTAL SINUS

The frontal sinuses are asymmetrical paired cavities located between the two tables of the frontal bone (Figure 6.1). The frontal sinuses are frequently divided by numerous incomplete bony septi into several intercommunicating air cells (Figure 6.2). The frontal air cells usually lie in the same coronal plane, but occasionally one sinus lies behind the other, in which case, it is referred to as a supernumerary frontal sinus. The frontal sinus is connected to the nasal cavity via the frontal recess.

The shape and size of the frontal sinus are highly variable, and it may be hypoplastic or even absent (Figure 6.3). On plain radiographs this anomaly may be misinterpreted as disease that has obliterated the sinus lumen. Computed tomographic (CT) evaluation of the sinuses with narrow window settings alone may also lead to misinterpretation of the under-developed sinus as a sinus exhibiting pathology. A wide- or bone-window setting will identify this as hypoplasia and exclude the possibility of a well-developed sinus with pathology affecting its lumen. Asymmetry of the frontal sinuses is more common in those races with dolichocephalic heads, such as the mongoloid race.

Extensive pneumatization of the superciliary portion of the frontal bone is a common variant in both normal individuals and acromegalics (Figure 6.4). It is not uncommon for this to be the only part of the frontal bone that is pneumatized and the normal supraorbital extension of the frontal sinus may be absent.

The anterior ethmoid air cells may encroach upon the frontal sinuses. These anterior ethmoid cells become clinically significant when they are so closely related to the frontal recess that they obstruct ventilation and drainage of the frontal sinus. This variant may be seen on the coronal scan as either a solitary air cell or a collection of air cells situated in the medial part of the floor of the frontal sinus, projecting into the lumen of the frontal sinus. These cells, which may also be referred to as a frontal bulla (Figure 6.5), usually drain into an already narrowed frontal recess.

THE FRONTAL RECESS

The term frontonasal duct is a misnomer, as this area has no duct-like features and is composed instead of a variably waisted hour-glass shaped bony channel through which the frontal sinus drains into the ostiomeatal complex. The frontal recess is rarely visualized at the time of routine, preoperative endoscopy, and CT in the coronal plane is ideal for assessing this region. A short, wide frontal recess may be easily visualized on a single scan. However, a more tortuous and narrow frontal recess usually cannot be seen on a single scan because the frontal recess runs obliquely with its distal (inferior) end more posterior than its proximal (superior) end.

The route of ventilation and drainage of the frontal sinus through the frontal recess depends upon the embryologic development as described in Chapter 3. The frontal recess may open into:

i   the premeatal groove anterior to the semilunar hiatus (Figure 6.6), and therefore drain independently of the ethmoid infundibulum and the maxillary and ethmoid sinuses;
ii   the ethmoid infundibulum; in this situation inflammation affecting the maxillary sinus may spread along the infundibulum to affect the frontal sinus.

The dimensions of the frontal recess are variable. If wide and short, the sinus is easily ventilated (Figure 6.7). However, if the frontal recess is long, tortuous and narrow and runs between crowded anterior ethmoid air cells, then minimal swelling can impede the drainage of the frontal sinus and predispose it to recurrent infection.

The frontal recess may be localized on CT or MR scans by identifying the superior insertion of the uncinate process (Figures 6.7–6.10; see also Figure 3.19). This superior insertion of the uncinate process is variable and determines whether the frontal recess drains into the ethmoid infundibulum or the premeatal groove. When the uncinate process inserts laterally into the lamina papyracea, the ethmoid infundibulum forms a blind recess, the terminal recess (recessus terminalis), and the frontal recess drains medially into the premeatal chamber of the ethmoid sinus (Figure 6.8). When the uncinate process inserts into the roof of the ethmoid sinus, or medially onto the middle turbinate, the frontal sinus drains directly into the ethmoid infundibulum (see Figure 3.19). The frontal recess may pneumatize the crista galli, middle turbinate or the agger nasi, and can thus both influence and be influenced by disease in these adjacent air cells.

Anatomic variants

The frontal recess may be obstructed by several anatomic variants, including enlarged agger nasi air cells, hypertrophied middle turbinates, concha bullosa or large anteriorly protruding ethmoid bulla. Deviations of the nasal septum may also narrow the frontal recess and the premeatal region of the ethmoid infundibulum.

THE AGGER NASI CELLS

CT in the coronal plane demonstrates the agger mound as a small prominence seen anterior and superior to the insertion of the vertical plate of the middle turbinate. When present, the agger nasi air cells are situated within the agger mound and are part of the anterior ethmoid sinuses (Figure 6.11). The agger mound may be acellular or it may contain between one and four air cells (Figure 6.12). Pneumatization of the agger mound may be so extensive that it encroaches either upon the lacrimal bone or upon the neck of the middle turbinate. Pneumatization of the agger mound can shorten the neck of the middle turbinate, resulting in a tight frontal recess (Figure 6.13).

Most agger nasi cells arise from, and are therefore aerated from, the frontal recess. The agger nasi cells are closely related to the lacrimal sac, being separated from the lacrimal sac by only the delicate lacrimal bone. This thin bony plate may be naturally dehiscent and as a result, inflammation can spread readily into the lacrimal sac, resulting in epiphora, dacryocystitis and sometimes preseptal or periorbital cellulitis.

DEVIATIONS OF THE NASAL SEPTUM

The nasal septum, which is almost never perfectly midline, is formed partly by the perpendicular plate of the ethmoid, the vomer, the palatine bones and the quadrilateral cartilage (Figures 6.3 and 6.14). While deviations of the nasal septum are common, not all deviations are of clinical significance. Most septal deviations are the result of developmental anomalies and asymmetric growth of the facial skeleton, although the nasal septum may deviate due to trauma. There may be a deviation of either the bony nasal septum, the cartilaginous septum or a combination of both (Figure 6.15).

Deviation of the nasal septum often allow compensatory hypertrophy of the contralateral inferior and sometimes the middle turbinate (Figure 6.15). A septal deviation may limit surgical access to the middle meatus, and a septoplasty may be required (Figure 6.16). Bony projections may extend laterally from the nasal septum. These bony spurs, (Figure 6.17) which vary in size, may be large enough to push into the lateral nasal wall, coming into contact with the middle or inferior turbinates or, in extreme cases, curling up into the middle meatus. Such contact may lead to severe headaches as well as nasal obstruction.

The nasal septum may be pneumatized, either in continuity with an aerated crista galli, or posteriorly as an extension of the sphenoid sinus (Figure 6.18).

Defects of the cartilaginous or bony septum with intact mucosa are usually the result of a previous submucous resection or septoplasty. Small perforations seen in the septum are most commonly the result of a previous septoplasty. Causes of larger cartilaginous traumatic septal hematomas, repeated local trauma, excessive cautery for epistaxis (chronic nose picking), midline granulomas (Stewart's or Wegener's), cocaine abuse, tuberculosis and leprosy. Atraumatic bony septal perforations are usually secondary to syphilis.

THE PNEUMATIZED CRISTA GALLI

The crista galli is the vertical extension of the perpendicular plate of the ethmoid bone above the cribriform plate into the anterior cranial cavity (Figure 6.11). The dura mater is attached to the crista galli. The crista galli may be pneumatized from the frontal recess and a large air cell may replace the entire body (Figure 6.8); it may be filled with fatty marrow (Figure 6.7). If the lumen of the air cell is narrow, it may become obstructed by minimal mucosal swelling. Patients with such an anomaly may present with headaches. In isolated frontal recess disease with secondary infection of a crista galli air cell, endoscopic and plain radiographic findings may be normal.

THE MAXILLARY SINUS

The maxillary sinuses are the largest of the paranasal sinuses. They are pyramidal shaped cavities, with the apex pointing towards the zygoma and the base forming the medial wall of the maxillary sinus. Most maxillary sinuses are symmetrical (Figures 6.6–6.8 and 6.10). CT in the coronal plane demonstrates the maxillary sinus to be narrow anteriorly, i.e. in the same plane as the vertical plate of the middle turbinate (Figure 6.19), widest in its midportion, i.e. in the same plane as the horizontal plate of the middle turbinate, and narrow again posteriorly.

The roof of the maxillary sinus forms the orbital floor which is narrow posteriorly and wider anteriorly. The inferior surface of the orbital floor is grooved by the infraorbital canal (Figure 6.19), which contains the infraorbital nerve as its accompanying vessels. This nerve passes through the infraorbital fissure (Figure 6.20), traverses the infraorbital canal and exits through the infraorbital foramen, which is situated below the inferior margin of the orbital rim (Figures 6.19–6.21). The bone surrounding the infraorbital nerve is usually thin and may be affected by erosion and reactive osteitis, with new bone formation in cases of chronic inflammatory sinus disease.

The posterior wall of the maxillary sinus is narrow and forms the anterior boundary of the pterygopalatine fossa (Figure 6.22). This region is better demonstrated by CT in the axial plane (see Figure 6.22).

The medial wall of the maxillary sinus forms part of the lateral wall of the nasal cavity. The bone of the medial wall is usually deficient over a large area, and the dehiscence is closed by the mucosa of both the nasal cavity and the maxillary sinus, covering a thin fibrous layer in continuation with the periosteum. This area is divided into the anterior and posterior nasal fontanelles. These latter two sections are separated by the ethmoid process of the inferior turbinate. These fontanelles should not be mistaken for bony erosion associated with disease. Small defects are frequently found in the membranous fontanelles; these are the accessory maxillary sinus ostia. They are usually situated immediately above the inferior turbinate and open directly into the middle meatus (Figure 6.20).

The maxillary sinus has three recesses: the alveolar recess, the lateral recess and the superior recess. The most frequently encountered recess is the alveolar recess, which is an inferior extension of the sinus into the alveolar ridge (Figure 6.23). Extension of the maxillary sinus into the zygoma is called the lateral recess of the maxillary sinus. The superior recess is the supermedial extension of the sinus, which can have a variable relationship to the orbit (Figures 6.24 and 6.25). The superior recess is well demonstrated by CT in the axial plane and may be mistaken for a large ethmoid air cell. The ethmoid sinus should be noted to be lying medially (Figure 6.25).

The maxillary sinus is separated from the posterior ethmoid sinus by the ethmomaxillary plate (Figures 6.20 and 6.21). Defects secondary to a previous transnasal ethmoidectomy may be seen in this plate.

Anatomic variants

Anatomic variants of the maxillary sinus that may be demonstrated by CT include asymmetry, hypoplasia of one or both maxillary sinuses, septated sinuses, a double maxillary sinus, an atelectatic maxillary sinus and an ethmomaxillary sinus.

Hypoplasia of the maxillary sinus

Hypoplasia of the maxillary sinus is a developmental abnormality that can be identified radiologically in patients with and without sinus disease. Bolger, Butzin and Parsons (1991) analyzed a series of 202 consecutively obtained CT scans, and noted an incidence of maxillary sinus hypoplasia of 10%. They presented a classification system based upon the radiographic features of the sinus as seen on CT. Type I maxillary sinus hypoplasia (incidence 7%) has only a mild degree of hypoplasia of the maxillary sinus, with a normal uncinate process and a normal infundibulum. Type II maxillary sinus hypoplasia (incidence 3%) has a mild to moderate reduction in the volume of the maxillary sinus, combined with CT evidence of a hypoplastic uncinate process and an absent or poorly defined infundibulum. In Type III maxillary sinus (incidence 0.5%), the maxillary sinus is largely absent and consists of only a cleft. The uncinate process is absent in Type III.

The nasal cavity and orbit on the involved side are usually enlarged. The maxillary sinus and the nasal cavity are inversely proportional to one another. The smaller the sinus, the larger the nasal cavity on the same side. The orbital rim may be at a lower level than the normal side with the eyeball appearing deeply placed, with an apparent 'exophthalmos' on the contralateral side. The sinus does not extend laterally as expected, and the infraorbital foramen appears to be more laterally placed (Figures 6.26

and 6.27). The pterygopalatine fossa and the superior and the inferior orbital fissures are enlarged, and the bony walls are thick. The natural ostium is bony.

In Type II maxillary sinus hypoplasia, there is marked retraction of the posterior fontanelle into the cavity of the maxillary sinus and the membranous fontanelle may be misdiagnosed as an air–fluid level (Figures 6.28 and 6.29). The uncinate process is fused with the inferomedial wall of the orbit.

Asymmetric sinuses may be demonstrated by plain radiographs. The smaller sinus may however be misinterpreted as a sinus of normal dimensions with chronic maxillary sinusitis, especially when the patient has a history of persistent upper respiratory tract infections. In such circumstances these patients may be erroneously subjected to prolonged medical management and may undergo surgical exploration only to find normal sinus mucosa within the smaller sinus cavity. The superior bone, air and soft-tissue contrast resolution of CT enables the radiologist to accurately diagnose such variants and has led to the finding of the association of hypoplasia of the uncinate process, with hypoplasia of the maxillary sinus. With increasing severity of the hypoplasia, a corresponding degree of hypoplasia or aplasia of the uncinate has been noted. This finding should be documented because an attempted uncinectomy in these patients will lead to inadvertent entry into the orbit through the lamina papyracea or orbital floor.

Hypoplasia of the maxillary sinus that is acquired following infection, trauma or radiation is represented by a maxilla of normal size, with the inflammatory reaction producing a partial or complete obliteration and resorption of the sinus lumen.

Atelectatic maxillary sinus

This anatomic variant may present as an asymptomatic incidental finding or in a patient with chronic sinusitis.

Maxillary sinus hyperplasia

Maxillary sinus hyperplasia is an uncommon condition in which there has been extensive pneumatization of the maxilla, with large recesses that pneumatize the alveolar ridge, and the zygoma (alveolar and lateral recesses). There is compensatory narrowing of the nasal cavity in these patients.

Septated maxillary sinus

The maxillary sinus may be subdivided by septi that may be either fibrous or bony and which divide the sinus into two unequal halves. These septi usually extend from the infraorbital canal to the lateral wall of the sinus, thereby forming a superolateral and an inferomedial compartment. Such anomalies should be identified to prevent incomplete drainage procedures which may result in the persistence of sinus disease (Figure 6.30).

Double maxillary sinus

This is a rare anomaly in which two independent cavities in the same maxilla drain into the middle meatus through two separate ostia.

Ethmomaxillary sinus

In this condition, the posterior ethmoid sinus extends laterally into the maxilla, forming an ethmo-maxillary sinus (Figure 6.31). This anomaly has the appearance of a septated sinus, but it can be differentiated by identifying the superior compartment which, having developed from the posterior ethmoid, drains into the superior meatus. The adjacent superior meatus is usually deeper and larger, whereas the related maxillary sinus is smaller or normal in size.

MAXILLARY SINUS OSTIUM

The natural ostium of the maxillary sinus is located in the superomedial aspect of the medial sinus wall. This natural ostium is radiographically located at the lateral end of the ethmoid infundibulum (the narrow channel lying between the lateral surface of the uncinate process, the lamina papyracea and the anterior surface of the ethmoid bulla). The ethmoid infundibulum opens through the semilunar hiatus into the middle meatus (Figure 6.19).

Anatomic variants

The accessory maxillary sinus ostia are small defects frequently found in the membranous anterior or posterior nasal fontanelles. These are situated immediately above the inferior turbinate and usually open directly into the anterior or posterior portions of the middle meatus (Figure 6.20). Accessory maxillary sinus ostia do not normally assist in the drainage of the maxillary sinus. They may be readily identified on endoscopy and may be misinterpreted as the true maxillary sinus ostium. The latter which opens into the depths of the ethmoid infundibulum is rarely visualized without resection of the uncinate process.

Because the maxillary sinus ostium is rarely seen during routine office endoscopy, it can be difficult to identify any anatomic variations that may be compromising the ventilation of this sinus and therefore predisposing the sinus to recurrent infections. Those common anomalies that may compromise the natural ostium include Haller's cells, lateral deviations of the uncinate process and a large ethmoid bulla. All of these anomalies which compromise the maxillary sinus ostium are best demonstrated by coronal CT.

HALLER'S CELLS

Haller's cells are named after the eighteenth-century anatomist, Albert von Haller, who described this particular anatomic variant. These cells are a lateral extension of the anterior ethmoid cells into the inferomedial margin of the orbit. Haller's cells cannot be seen on endoscopic examination of the nasal cavity, however they are clearly demonstrated by CT in the coronal plane (Figure 6.32). A solitary large Haller's cell situated lateral to the maxillary sinus ostium may narrow the lumen and predispose the sinus to recurrent infections. The pneumatization of the floor of the orbit by Haller's cells may be extensive (Figure 6.33).

THE ETHMOID SINUS

The ethmoid bone lies between the orbits. It is comprised of a horizontal plate, a vertical plate and, on either side of the latter, the ethmoid labyrinths (Figures 6.19, 6.25 and 6.34–6.37). The ethmoid labyrinth is separated from the orbit by the delicate lamina papyracea. Natural dehiscences in the lamina papyracea may serve as small channels allowing the spread of infection into the orbit. These findings should not be misinterpreted as pathologic erosions.

The vertical plate extends above the horizontal cribriform plate into the anterior cranial fossa as the crista galli. The horizontal plate of the ethmoid is perforated for the transmission of the olfactory nerve fibers from the roof of the nasal cavity (Figure 6.38). The gyrus rectus of the frontal lobe and the olfactory bulb rest upon the olfactory fossa on either side of the crista galli.

The cribriform plate lies at a variable level in relation to the ethmoid foveolae. It may lie well below the roof of the ethmoid or, in some cases, in the same plane as the ethmoid foveolae (Figures 6.35 and 6.38). This is well demonstrated on CT in the coronal plane. If sinus surgery is being contemplated, the surgeon will use this information to avoid injury to the cribriform plate. Such injuries may be complicated by permanent anosmia or cerebrospinal fluid rhinorrhea and the risk of intracranial infection.

The ethmoid labyrinths are divided into an anterior and a posterior group of air cells (see Figure 6.37). The ground lamella of the middle turbinate is the dividing line between the anterior and the posterior ethmoid cells. The anterior ethmoid air cells are usually smaller and more numerous than the posterior group of air cells. The anterior ethmoid cells drain into the middle meatus whereas the posterior ethmoid cells drain into the superior meatus.

The anterior ethmoid sinuses

The anatomy of the anterior ethmoid sinus is variable. These variations are of clinical interest when they cause obstruction of the ostiomeatal complex. The ostiomeatal complex is the key to the development of most inflammatory diseases of the frontal, maxillary and ethmoid sinuses.

The ostiomeatal complex is a term used to collectively describe that area of the anterior ethmoid into which the frontal, the maxillary, and the anterior ethmoidal sinuses drain. The ostiomeatal complex is comprised of the frontal recess, the infundibulum, the semilunar hiatus and the adjacent portion of the middle meatus. Anatomically, this area is bounded by the medial wall of the maxillary sinus and the lamina papyracea laterally, the lateral surface of the uncinate process anteriorly and medially, and the anterior wall of the ethmoid bulla posteriorly (Figures 6.6, 6.8 and 6.19).

The ethmoid bulla

The largest and most constantly present anterior ethmoid air cell is the ethmoid bulla. The ethmoid bulla is the most prominent structure seen clinically when the middle turbinate is retracted medially (Figure 6.39). The anterior wall of the ethmoid bulla forms the posterior margin of the ethmoid infundibulum. The roof of the ethmoid bulla may be continuous with the roof of the ethmoid sinus or it may be separated by a suprabullar extension of the lateral sinus. The ethmoid bulla is variable in its pneumatization. It may be absent or it may be expanded, inferiorly, medially or anteriorly, narrowing the middle meatus. If the ethmoid bulla expands medially it may make contact with the adjacent lateral surface of the middle turbinate, resulting in facial pain and contact headaches (Figure 6.40). If the ethmoid bulla enlarges anteroinferiorly it may overhang the semilunar hiatus and occlude the ethmoid infundibulum, thus obstructing its narrow drainage pathway (Figures 6.39 and 6.41). The frontal recess may be occluded by an ethmoid bulla that expands anteriorly. The ethmoid bulla often appears to have no mucosal disease, but it may be responsible for inflammatory disease in the neighboring larger paranasal sinuses (Figure 6.42).

THE UNCINATE PROCESS

The uncinate process forms the anterior and medial walls of the ethmoid infundibulum. The posterior free margin of the uncinate process forms the anterior border of the semilunar hiatus. The uncinate process of the ethmoid bone extends inferiorly to fuse with the ethmoidal process of the inferior turbinate (Figure 6.19). This fusion is usually at least 1 cm posterior to the distal end of the nasolacrimal duct. However, it is not uncommon to see this area of fusion quite close to the nasolacrimal duct (Figures 6.24 and 6.35). This observation should alert the surgeon to the risk of injury to the nasolacrimal apparatus because a generous uncinate resection may result in chronic epiphora if the nasolacrimal duct is transected. With such an anomaly the ethmoid infundibulum extends more anteriorly and disease in this area may affect the nasolacrimal apparatus, especially the more distal duct which has a membranous wall. The superior insertion of the uncinate process is variable. It may turn laterally to insert into the lamina papyracea or it may insert superiorly into the roof of the ethmoid (Figure 6.43; see also Figure 3.19). In some instances the uncinate process turns medially and inserts into the vertical plate of the middle turbinate (Figures 6.26 and 6.44), as discussed in the section on anatomic variations of the frontal recess.

Various anomalies of the uncinate process can occur. Rarely the uncinate process is hypoplastic. This anomaly has been associated with hypoplasia of the maxillary sinus and with the atelectatic maxillary sinus. In the latter condition, the middle meatus is wide and the posterior fontanelle retracted into the cavity of the maxillary sinus. The uncinate process appears to be 'plastered' to the inferomedial wall of the orbit, and attempted uncinectomy will inevitably lead to orbital injury (Figure 6.28).

The uncinate process may be medially deviated, causing obstruction of the middle meatus (Figures 6.44 and 6.45). It may instead deviate laterally, causing obstruction of the ethmoid infundibulum and the maxillary sinus ostium (Figure 6.39). Should the posterior free margin of the uncinate process be deflected medially, it may resemble a turbinate and has, in this position, been incorrectly referred to as an accessory or double middle turbinate (Figure 6.46). The uncinate process may protrude anteriorly and compromise the middle meatus.

Occasionally the uncinate process is pneumatized. This air cell may be large enough to occlude the ethmoid infundibulum (Figure 6.47), or it may even be the site of polyp formation. The uncinate process may also be hypertrophied (Figures 6.48 and 6.49).

THE ETHMOID INFUNDIBULUM

This critical drainage channel is bordered by the uncinate process anteromedially, the anterior surface of the ethmoid bulla posteriorly and the lamina papyracea laterally (Figure 6.19). The ethmoid infundibulum connects the natural ostium of the maxillary sinus to the middle meatus via the semilunar hiatus. Variations in the anatomy of the related structures that border the ethmoid infundibulum, i.e. the uncinate process and the ethmoid bulla, can result in permanent narrowing or intermittent obstruction of this channel (Figure 6.41). The ethmoid infundibulum may also be compromised by anomalies of the middle turbinate (Figure 6.50). Anteriorly and superiorly, the frontal recess may open into the ethmoid infundibulum. Posteriorly,

when present, the lateral sinus, which lies between the ethmoid bulla and the basal lamella, also opens via the semilunar hiatus into the ethmoid infundibulum.

The semilunar hiatus

The semilunar hiatus is a semilunar two-dimensional aperture bounded posteriorly by the anterior surface of the ethmoid bulla and anteriorly by the posterior free margin of the uncinate process (Figure 6.19). It is the opening through which the ethmoid infundibulum drains into the middle meatus.

The lateral sinus (recess) and the basal lamella

The basal lamella of the middle turbinate is the septum that divides the anterior from the posterior ethmoid sinuses. The lateral sinus is an inconstant space that lies between the ethmoid bulla and the basal lamella (see Figure 3.18). The lateral sinus can extend above the bulla and thus create a supra bullar space (Figure 6.51). The lateral recess opens directly into the posterosuperior part of the semilunar hiatus and is sometimes referred to as the superior recess of the semilunar hiatus. A large ethmoid bulla overhanging this aperture or a swollen medially bent uncinate process can impede the drainage of the lateral recess into the middle meatus. The radiologist must be able to identify the lateral sinus, as inflammatory disease may be confined to the lateral sinus and only identifiable on CT scan.

THE MIDDLE TURBINATE AND MIDDLE MEATUS

The middle meatus

The middle meatus is the space inferolateral to the middle turbinate, into which the anterior ethmoid, the frontal and the maxillary sinuses eventually drain (Figures 6.19 and 6.21). The middle meatus can be more clearly seen by medial retraction of the middle turbinate during endoscopy. The most prominent structure within the middle meatus is usually the ethmoid bulla. The uncinate process lies anterior to the ethmoid bulla. The size of the middle meatus can vary; for example, it may be deep when the maxillary sinus is atelectatic and the posterior fontanelle is retracted laterally (Figures 6.28 and 6.29). The middle meatus and the nasal cavities are small when the sinuses are well developed.

Anatomic variants

The middle meatus may be compromised by a large ethmoid bulla, a deviated nasal septum, a bony septal spur or one of the many variants of the middle turbinates (such as an abnormally aerated middle turbinate – a concha bullosa), a secondary middle turbinate or an accessory middle turbinate.

'Accessory middle turbinate'

When the free posterior margin of the uncinate process deflects medially it resembles a Mexican hat and may be incorrectly identified clinically as an accessory or double middle turbinate (Figures 6.46 and 6.52). This anomaly may cause mucosal apposition, which subsequently leads to inflammatory changes and polypoidal degeneration. The accessory middle turbinate may be mistaken for a polyp on casual examination.

Deviated nasal septum

Deviations of the cartilaginous or bony parts, or both, of the nasal septum may obstruct the nasal cavity. Contact between the opposing mucosal surfaces can cause headaches and may be the site of polypoidal degeneration of the mucosa. Septal deviations are well demonstrated by CT and a wider perspective may be gained of the influence of bony spurs on the nasal cavity. This is of great clinical value because it may be extremely difficult to assess the nasal cavity beyond a marked deviation or spur (see earlier section deviations of the nasal septum).

Secondary middle turbinate

Rarely, a small secondary turbinate is seen in the middle meatus (Figure 6.52). This is comprised of

bone covered by soft tissue and projects medially from the lateral nasal wall into the middle meatus before turning superiorly within the meatus to appear as an inverted turbinate. This anomaly has not been noted to compromise the ostiomeatal complex. A secondary middle turbinate should not be confused with a medially bent uncinate process, also called an 'accessory middle turbinate', nor should it be mistaken for a polyp.

The middle turbinate

The middle turbinate arises from the medial aspect of the ethmoid labyrinth. Anteriorly, the middle turbinate is suspended from the roof of the ethmoid by a vertical bony plate (Figures 6.10, 6.34, 6.35 and 6.38). The vertical plate of the middle turbinate serves as an important anatomic landmark for the cribriform plate during intranasal surgery and should not be resected, in case revision surgery is required in the future. The head of the middle turbinate is slightly bulbous in shape and is continuous posteriorly with the free margin of the middle turbinate. The head usually protrudes anterior to the vertical plate by 1–2 mm, although it may protrude by over 1 cm. It is therefore an unreliable landmark for the uncinate process.

Several thin inconstant plates may be seen arising from the middle turbinate and insert laterally on to the lamina papyracea. The largest and most constant of these horizontal plates curves laterally to insert on to the lamina papyracea (Figures 6.20 and 6.46), and forms the roof of the middle meatus. This is referred to as the basal or ground lamella, which separates the anterior ethmoid sinuses from the posterior ethmoid sinuses.

The free margin of the middle turbinate is usually bulbous but it can be triangular or bifid or have a sagittal groove which incompletely divides it into unequal parts (Figures 6.28 and 6.53).

Anatomic variants

The advent of CT has advanced our understanding of the variations that occur in the middle turbinate. These anatomic variants are readily identified by CT and include aeration of the middle turbinate (a concha bullosa), hypertrophy of the middle turbinate, paradoxically bent middle turbinate, lateralization of the turbinate, bony hypertrophy of the middle turbinate (Figure 6.54), and partial or complete agenesis (Figure 6.49).

Concha bullosa: aeration of the middle turbinate

The middle turbinates may be pneumatized from the ethmoid sinuses or directly from the middle meatus. An air cell in a middle turbinate is called a concha bullosa (Figures 6.50 and 6.55). The incidence of concha bullosa is approximately 24%, and it may be unilateral or bilateral. The pneumatization of a concha bullosa is usually from the frontal recess, from a lateral sinus or from the agger nasi, but occasionally it is directly from the nasal cavity. Not all conchae bullosae cause symptoms, and they may simply be an incidental radiographic finding. A concha bullosa becomes of clinical significance when it is large enough to compress the ethmoid infundibulum, obstruct the nasal cavity or cause lateral displacement of the uncinate process. Such patients present with sinugenic headaches or recurrent sinusitis (Figure 6.50).

The air cell may be confined to the free margin, the vertical plate, or the horizontal plate of the middle turbinate. In some instances, the entire middle turbinate may be pneumatized. The superior meatus may extend into the vertical plate of the middle turbinate. This particular type of air cell is referred to as an 'interlamellar cell'. There may be more than one interlamellar cell (up to three) (Figure 6.56). The middle meatus may be narrowed by large concha bullosa, and an anteriorly protruding concha may obstruct the frontal recess (see Figure 7.8). If this occurs, then there will usually be an increased incidence of inflammatory disease of the associated neighboring paranasal sinuses (Figure 6.55).

In the asymptomatic phase, CTs may demonstrate early mucosal apposition between a concha bullosa and the adjacent structures. A large concha bullosa may appear to cause a secondary deflection of the nasal septum to the opposite side, and the contralateral middle turbinate may be small or paradoxically bent (Figure 6.50).

The small cleft between the ethmoid bulla laterally, and the middle turbinate medially, is called the conchal or turbinate sinus. Here the adjacent mucosa may make contact if any one of these structures is enlarged. Prolonged contact results in inflammatory changes in this space, with or without polypoidal degeneration. This is one of the commonest sites for polyp formation (Figure 6.40).

Paradoxically bent middle turbinate

Normally the lateral surface of the middle turbinate is concave, curving away from the lateral nasal wall to allow space for the middle meatus. When the lateral surface of the middle turbinate is convex or the turbinate appears to be bending medially, it is called a paradoxically bent middle turbinate (Figure 6.50). This usually occurs bilaterally and may reduce the middle meatus considerably. A concha bullosa occurring in a paradoxically bent middle turbinate may further reduce the middle meatus and thus contribute to the pathogenesis of sinus disease.

Lateralized middle turbinate

A lateralized middle turbinate is an unusually small turbinate that is laterally placed, resulting in contact with the adjacent uncinate process. It may obstruct the ethmoid infundibulum (Figure 6.57).

Hypertrophied middle turbinate

On routine clinical examination it is not possible to differentiate between a hypertrophied and a pneumatized middle turbinate. However, the difference becomes apparent on examination of CTs. The hypertrophy may be of either soft tissue (Figure 6.58) or bone (Figure 6.54).

THE INFERIOR TURBINATE AND INFERIOR MEATUS

The anterior end of the inferior turbinate and the inferior meatus are the first structures that are seen on clinical examination of the nasal cavity. The inferior turbinate is an independent bone that fuses laterally with the conchal ridge of the medial process of the maxilla. The inferior meatus lies inferolateral to the inferior turbinate and the nasolacrimal duct is the only structure that opens into this meatus (Figures 6.8, 6.19, 6.22 and 6.59).

The mucous membrane of the inferior turbinate contains erectile tissue, the dilatation of which may be responsible for much of the soft-tissue hypertrophy. A marked reduction in the size of the inferior turbinate may be noted following the application of a topical vasoconstrictor such as 0.1% xylometazoline hydrochloride nasal solution, thus indicating that such patients may benefit from cauterization or a limited turbinectomy (Figures 6.60 and 6.61). Irreversible hypertrophy of the inferior turbinates may be indicative of vasomotor rhinitis or allergic rhinitis.

Preoperative CT is rarely indicated to assess hypertrophy of the inferior turbinates. However, if there is suspicion of ethmoid sinus disease causing secondary inferior turbinate vasodilatation, or the presence of a large bony inferior turbinate causing obstruction, then the ethmoid sinus disease or the bony abnormality can be well demonstrated by CT. Submucosal resection of the enlarged bony portion of the inferior turbinate bone may be curative (Figure 6.62). Soft-tissue hypertrophy of the inferior turbinate is much commoner than bony hypertrophy and is also easily demonstrable (Figures 6.15 and 6.63). An uncommon cause for enlargement of the inferior turbinate is pneumatization of the turbinate bone. This is an unusual finding and the pneumatization is usually derived from the maxillary sinus (Figure 6.64).

The posterior ethmoid sinuses

The posterior ethmoid air cells are larger in size than the anterior ethmoid air cells, but fewer in number. They drain into the superior meatus, which is situated inferolateral to the superior turbinate. An inconstant additional turbinate may be situated above the superior turbinate and is called the supreme turbinate (Figures 6.38 and 6.46). The largest and most posterior of the posterior ethmoid air cells is called Onodi's cell, after the anatomist who first described it, when it exposes a lateral bulging of the optic canal, a so-called 'tuberculum opticum'. Onodi's cell shares a common wall with the adjacent sphenoid sinus and is best demonstrated by CT in the axial plane (Figure 6.36).

Onodi's cells are of great clinical importance as they have an intimate relationship with the optic nerve, from which they are separated by a thin delicate bony septa. It is not uncommon for the bone to be dehiscent in this region and it is of critical importance that the relationship of the optic nerve to the posterior ethmoid is identified, in order to avoid injury to the optic nerve and blindness.

The pneumatization of the posterior ethmoids is variable and it is not uncommon for the posterior ethmoid sinuses to extend beyond the confines of the ethmoid bone. The posterior ethmoid may expand superiorly into the orbit forming supraorbital cells, or it may expand laterally to encompass the optic nerve. These variants, if not identified preoperatively, pose extreme hazards to the patient's vision.

The lateral extension of the posterior ethmoid into the maxilla is called the ethmomaxillary sinus and has already been discussed. Another variant is the lateral and posterior extension of the ethmoid air cells around the sphenoid sinus on either side. This variant is referred to as the ethmosphenoid sinus. The ethmosphenoid sinus is clinically important because of the structures related to the lateral wall of the sphenoid sinus, especially the internal carotid artery which may have a close relation to the posterior ethmoid sinus. Surgical intervention is more common in the posterior ethmoid sinus than the sphenoid and, in the posterior ethmoid, the internal carotid artery may only be separated from the sinus by a thin plate of bone.

Irrespective of the bone that is pneumatized by these ethmoids, all these additional air cells drain into the posterior ethmoid sinus and superior meatus (Figure 6.31).

THE SPHENOID SINUS

The sphenoid is a complex bone with several processes. The lesser wing and the anterior clinoid process are attached anteriorly to the planum sphenoidale (Figure 6.65). The anterior clinoid process houses the canal of the optic nerve and also forms the superior margin of the superior orbital fissure. The superomedial aspect of the superior orbital fissure is separated from the optic nerve canal by a thin piece of bone called the optic strut (Figure 6.66). The greater wing of the sphenoid is situated more inferiorly and forms part of the orbital wall and the inferior margin of the superior orbital fissure. The pterygoid processes arise from the greater wing of the sphenoid and form the posterior border of the pterygopalatine fossa (Figures 6.22, 6.67 and 6.68). The greater wing of the sphenoid makes a major contribution to the anteromedial part of the middle cranial fossa (Figure 6.65). The foramen rotundum and the pterygoid (vidian) canal traverse the body of the sphenoid and are lateral relations of the sphenoid sinus (Figures 6.24, 6.66 and 6.67). Posteriorly, the foramen ovale and foramen spinosum perforate the greater wing close to the petrous apex (Figure 6.24).

The sphenoid sinuses are asymmetrical and vary in size. Superiorly the sphenoid sinus is related to the pituitary fossa and the pituitary gland (Figures 6.14 and 6.36). On either side of the sinus lie the cavernous sinuses which transmit the internal carotid artery and the third, fourth and sixth cranial nerves. The intracavernous portion of the internal carotid artery passes superiorly alongside the body of the sphenoid sinus (Figure 6.68). It comes to lie medial to the anterior clinoid process before perforating the dura, which roofs the cavernous sinus, and then becomes the terminal or cerebral part of the artery (Figures 6.24, 6.25, 6.36 and 6.69). The internal carotid artery may sometimes lie within the lumen of the sphenoid sinus. It is usually separated by a thin plate of bone, but this may be dehiscent. Inferiorly, the sphenoid sinus is related to the nasopharynx, the eustachian tubes and eustachian cushions (Figures 6.23 and 6.69).

Plain lateral radiographs of the skull demonstrate the sphenoid sinus well, but the adjacent structures related to the lateral wall of the sphenoid sinus are poorly demonstrated by the Caldwell view. Several anatomic variations occur in the sphenoid sinus, and these are well demonstrated by CT. It is not uncommon to find a multiseptate sinus (Figure 6.66). Several pneumatized recesses extend from the sinus into the surrounding structures. The commonest is the lateral recess that when present passes between the pterygoid (vidian) canal and the foramen rotundum (Figure 6.66). In some instances, the entire greater wing of the sphenoid bone, which makes a major contribution to the floor of the middle cranial fossa, is pneumatized. The anterior clinoid, the lesser wing of the sphenoid, the dorsum sella and sometimes the posterior clinoid process may be pneumatized. The sinus may also extend into the pterygoid processes. The floor of the sphenoid sinus may be dehiscent. This finding should not be misinterpreted as the natural ostium of the sinus (Figures 6.70 and 6.71). The dehiscence may be further eroded by benign or malignant disease. This is well demonstrated by CT in the coronal plane.

The sphenoid sinus drains through a small ostium in the anterior wall, close to the roof of the sinus, into the sphenoethmoid recess. This is usually not well demonstrated by CT in the coronal plane, but it is well demonstrated on scans taken in the axial plane or following sagittal reformation of images taken in the axial plane (Figure 6.36).

THE PTERYGOPALATINE FOSSA

The pterygopalatine fossa is shaped like an inverted pyramid bounded anteriorly by the maxillary sinus, medially by the palatine bone and posteriorly by the pterygoid plates of the sphenoid bone (Figures 6.22, 6.25 and 6.26). The pterygopalatine fossa communicates with the orbit, the nasopharynx, the paranasal sinuses, the infratemporal fossa and the middle cranial fossa, and it may form a major channel for the spread of infection or tumor. The contents of the fossa include the terminal branches of the maxillary artery, accompanying small veins, the maxillary nerve and the pterygopalatine ganglion, which transmits the parasympathetic nerve supply to the lacrimal gland, nasal cavity and nasopharynx. All of these structures are surrounded by loose connective tissue and fat. CT does not clearly demonstrate the contents of the pterygopalatine fossa, but following the administration of intravenous contrast the terminal branches of the maxillary artery may be seen as small enhancing structures. Obliteration of the fat spaces in the pterygopalatine fossa is indicative of disease, the commonest being malignancy invading the space.

The pterygopalatine fossa communicates directly with many of the surrounding anatomic regions, and these channels may be identified by CT. Posteriorly, the pterygopalatine fossa communicates with the middle cranial fossa via the foramen rotundum, which transmits the maxillary nerve (Figure 6.72). Inferiorly, the pterygopalatine fossa tapers to its apex and receives the pterygoid (vidian) canal. This canal passes anteriorly through the body of the sphenoid from the foramen lacerum and transmits the vidian nerve (Figure 6.24). The pterygopalatine fossa communicates with the oral cavity through the greater and lesser palatine canals (Figures 6.23 and 6.50), and laterally with the infra temporal fossa, containing the medial and lateral pterygoids via the pterygomaxillary fissure (Figures 6.24 and 6.73). Medially, it communicates through the sphenopalatine foramen with the sphenoethmoid recess and the nasal cavity (Figure 6.73). Anterosuperiorly, it communicates with the orbit through the infraorbital fissure (Figures 6.24 and 6.25).

THE ORBITAL APEX

The orbit is the bony cavity that houses the eyeball, extraocular muscles and neurovascular structures, including the optic nerve. The apex of the orbit communicates through the optic canal, the superior orbital fissure and the inferior orbital fissure with the middle cranial fossa, the pterygopalatine fossa and the inferior temporal fossa, respectively (Figure 6.74).

The optic canal traverses the lesser wing of the sphenoid bone, between the middle cranial fossa and the orbit, and transmits the optic nerve and the ophthalmic artery (Figure 6.65). Medially, the optic canal and nerve are separated from the posterior ethmoid and sphenoid sinuses by the lamina papyracea and a small part of the lesser wing of the sphenoid. Inferolaterally the optic canal and nerve are separated from the superior orbital fissure by a spicule of bone, called the optic strut, which is the root of the lesser wing of the sphenoid (Figure 6.65). The optic nerve is surrounded by a prolongation of the meninges. The ophthalmic artery usually lies inferior to the optic nerve.

The superior orbital fissure lies obliquely between the greater and the lesser wing of the sphenoid (Figures 6.36 and 6.65), and transmits the third, fourth and sixth cranial nerves, as well as the ophthalmic division of the fifth cranial nerve and the superior ophthalmic vein. A tendinous ring surrounds the medial aspect of the superior orbital fissure and the optic canal and gives origin to the four rectus muscles (Figures 6.75–6.77).

The infraorbital fissure transmits the infraorbital nerve and is the main communication between the orbit and both the pterygopalatine fossa and the infratemporal fossa (Figures 6.24, 6.25 and 6.74).

CTs of the orbital apex usually demonstrate these anatomic features clearly separated by fat. If the fat planes are obscured this may indicate early infiltration by tumor or aggressive infection. The tendinous ring giving origin to the rectus muscles occasionally shows enhancement following the administration of intravenous contrast and should not be mistaken for tumor.

THE LACRIMAL SAC AND NASOLACRIMAL DUCT

The nasolacrimal apparatus consists of the lacrimal gland situated in the superolateral aspect of the orbit, the lacrimal sac and the nasolacrimal duct. The lacrimal sac and the nasolacrimal duct are the final drainage pathways for the tears produced by the lacrimal gland. The lacrimal sac is a membranous sac situated in the lacrimal fossa inferolateral to the medial canthus. The lacrimal fossa is bounded anteriorly by the anterior lacrimal crest of the frontal process of the maxilla and posteriorly by the posterior lacrimal crest, which is a ridge on the lacrimal bone (Figure 6.13 and 6.25). The lacrimal sac has a bulbous fundus superiorly. Inferiorly, it tapers to become continuous with the nasolacrimal duct.

The nasolacrimal duct has two parts, intraosseous and membranous parts. It is directed inferiorly, posteriorly and slightly laterally. The intraosseous part is bounded by the maxilla, the lacrimal bone and the inferior turbinate (Figures 6.12 and 6.78). The nasolacrimal duct is narrowest in the middle (Figure 6.72). Inferiorly, it lies beneath the nasal mucosa and opens into the highest point of the inferior meatus, where it is protected by the Hasner's valve.

The lacrimal fossa is readily identified by CT in both the axial and coronal planes as a small impression in the inferomedial orbital wall. The lacrimal sac is usually seen as a soft-tissue density in the lacrimal fossa (Figure 6.13). It may be air-filled on occasions and should not be mistaken for orbital emphysema (Figure 6.79).

The membranous part of the nasolacrimal duct varies in its relationship to the base of the uncinate process and the ethmoidal infundibulum. This relationship should be identified prior to any surgery in this region. The nasolacrimal duct may be injured by a generous uncinectomy conducted during an endoscopic procedure (Figures 6.24 and 6.33), or by an excessive resection of the anterior margin of the natural ostium of the maxillary sinus. If the inferior turbinate is resected close to the base, the duct may be injured, resulting in permanent occlusion of the nasolacrimal canal and epiphora. The nasolacrimal duct may also become obstructed by inflammatory disease, trauma or neoplastic processes.

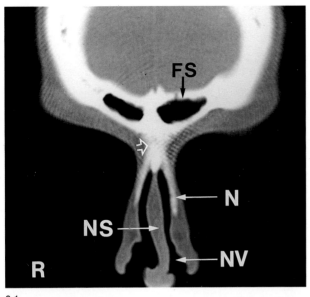

6.1

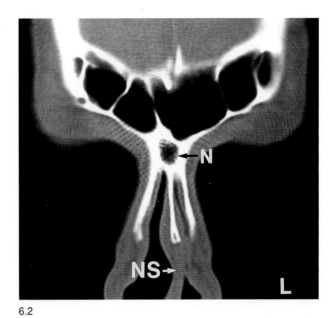

6.2

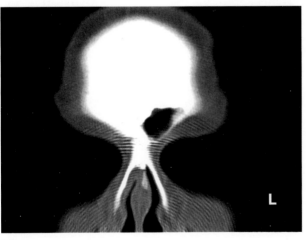

6.3

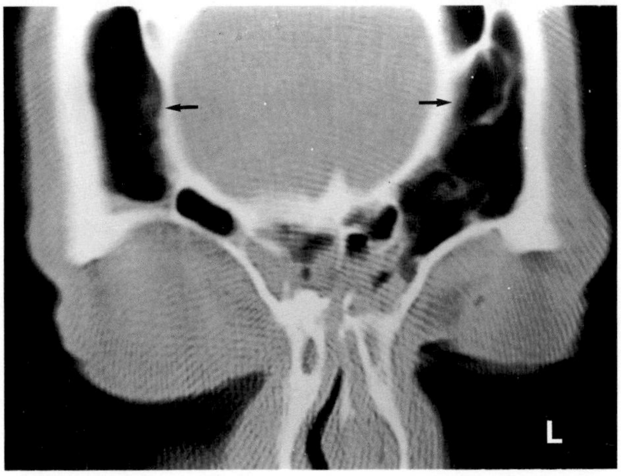

6.4

Figure **6.1**

The nasal pyramid. This anterior coronal CT scan cuts through the external nose and the most anterior portion of the frontal sinus. The frontal sinus (FS), the frontal process of the maxilla (N), the nasal bones (open arrow), the cartilaginous portion of the nasal septum (NS) and the nasal vestibule (NV).

Figure **6.2**

Septation of a normal frontal sinus. This coronal CT scan of the frontal sinuses demonstrates a multiseptated frontal sinus, normal nasal bones and an anterior deviation of the cartilaginous nasal septum (NS) to the left. Note the nasal cell (N) which, if extensive, may compromise the frontal recess.

Figure **6.3**

Aplasia of the right frontal sinus (CT). This is a common anomaly where one of the frontal sinuses is partially or completely undeveloped.

Figure **6.4**

Extensive pneumatization of the frontal sinus. This coronal CT scan of the frontal sinuses demonstrates extensive pneumatization of the frontal bone (arrows). In this case the anterior ethmoid air cells narrow the frontal recess and contain diseased mucosa. These anterior ethmoid cells are characteristically located along the floor of the frontal sinus, close to the midline.

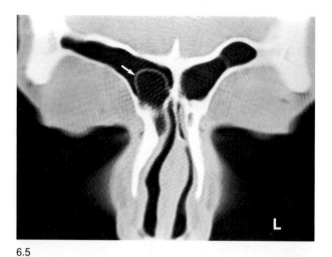

6.5

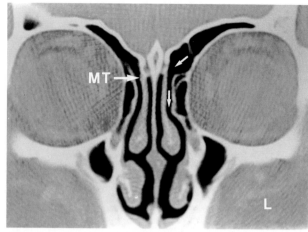

6.6

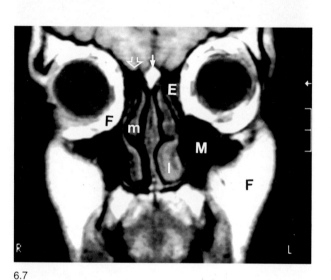

6.7

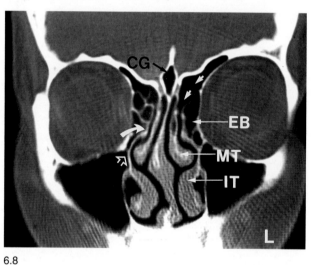

6.8

Figure **6.5**

A frontal bulla. This anterior CT scan through the frontal sinus demonstrates a small, anteriorly placed ethmoid air cell projecting into the floor of the frontal sinus (arrow). This is called a frontal bulla.

Figure **6.6**

CT of the normal frontal recess. This scan demonstrates a normal, wide, patent frontal recess (upper arrow). In this patient, the frontal recess drains directly into the middle meatus (lower arrow). The vertical insertion of the middle turbinate (MT) can be clearly seen.

Figure **6.7**

MR of the normal maxillary and ethmoid sinuses. This T1-weighted anterior coronal MR scan demonstrates the maxillary sinuses (M) and the ethmoid sinuses (E) as signal void (dark) spaces. The middle turbinate (m) and the inferior turbinate (I) are isointense with muscle. The bright signals in the orbits and cheeks (F) are due to fat. The bright midline signal is the result of fat in the crista galli (arrow). This scan demonstrates the intimate relationship of the frontal lobes to the ethmoid fovea (open arrow).

Figure **6.8**

Normal frontal recess (CT). A wide frontal recess is seen (arrows). The crista galli is pneumatized (CG). The ethmoid bulla (EB), and the middle (MT) and inferior turbinates (IT) are demonstrated. Inferior and lateral to the turbinates are the corresponding meati. The uncinate process attaches medially to the anterior ethmoid air cells (curved arrows). The right maxillary ostium is also demonstrated (open arrow) opening into the ethmoid infundibulum.

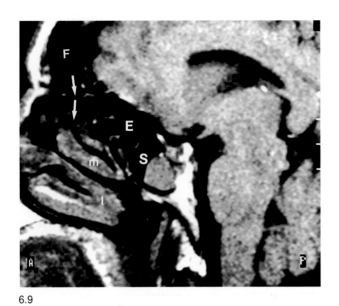

6.9

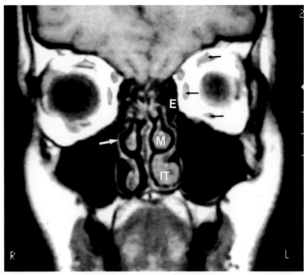

6.10

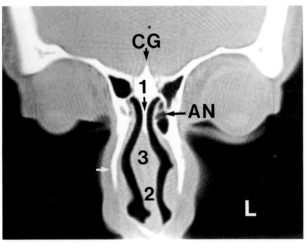

6.11

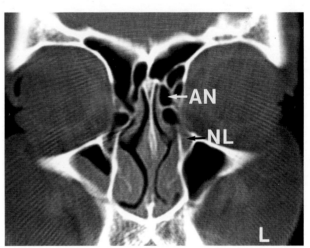

6.12

Figure 6.9

Sagittal MR scan through the frontal sinus. This T1-weighted MR scan demonstrates a normal frontal sinus (F) draining into the frontal recess (arrows). The other structures seen are the inferior turbinate (I), the middle turbinate (m), the ethmoid labyrinth (E) and a polyp in the sphenoid sinus (S).

Figure 6.11

Agger nasi cells. This coronal CT scan shows an agger nasi cell (AN). The right agger mound is acellular. Note the nasal septum formed superiorly by the perpendicular plate of the ethmoid bone (1), the cartilaginous portion of the nasal septum (the quadrilateral cartilage) (2). The localized expansion at the junction of the bony and cartilaginous portion of the nasal septum is the body of Zuckerkandl (3), which represents the vestigial remnants of erectile tissue. The frontal process of the maxilla (white arrow) and the crista galli (CG) are also shown.

Figure 6.10

Normal MR scan through the middle of the maxillary sinus. This T1-weighted scan demonstrates the middle (M), inferior (IT) and superior turbinates. The intraorbital muscles (black arrows) are well seen in the bright hyperintense intraorbital fat. The ethmoid sinus (E) and the uncinate process (white arrow); the lamina papyracea and the air in the ethmoid sinuses appear as signal void areas against the bright orbital fat.

Figure 6.12

CT of multiple agger nasi cells. The agger mound may be acellular or it may contain between one and seven air cells (AN). The nasolacrimal duct (NL) is also demonstrated.

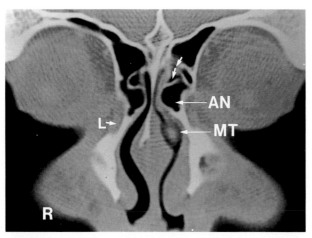

6.13

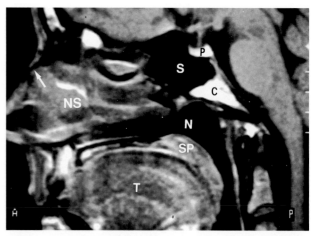

6.14

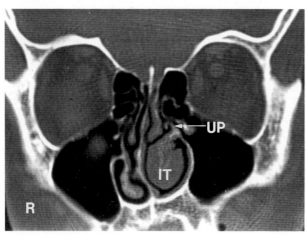

6.15

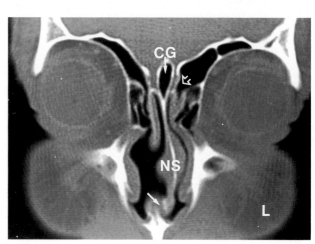

6.16

Figure **6.13**

CT demonstrating a large agger nasi cell (AN) occluding the frontal recess (arrows). The larger the agger nasi cell, the greater the encroachment on the neck of the middle turbinate (MT), resulting in a restricted frontal recess. The normal lacrimal fossa (L) is seen on the right side.

Figure **6.14**

Normal sagittal MR scan of the sphenoid sinus. This sagittal T1-weighted scan demonstrates the normal nasal septum (NS), the sphenoid sinus (S), the pituitary gland and its stalk (P), the nasal bone (arrow), the soft palate (SP), the tongue (T), the nasopharynx (N) and the clivus (C), which is hyperintense due to its fatty marrow.

Figure **6.15**

Deviated nasal septum. This CT scan shows a deviation of the nasal septum to the right. There is compensatory hypertrophy of the left inferior turbinate (IT), and a paradoxically bent, hypoplastic right inferior turbinate. The left uncinate process (UP) is curved and bends inferiorly.

Figure **6.16**

Post-traumatic nasal septal deviation. The nasal septum (NS) is seen deviated to the left. The left frontal recess (open arrow) would be difficult to approach without a prior septoplasty. The deviation of the nasal septum was the result of trauma. Note the fractureline at the base of the septum (arrow). The crista galli is aerated (CG).

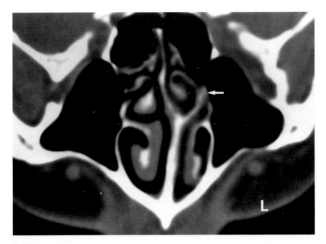

6.17

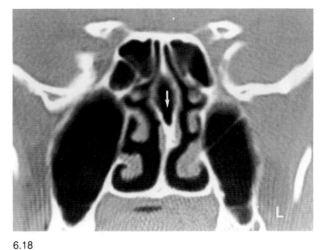

6.18

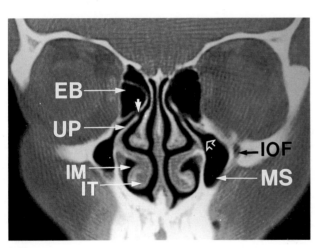

6.19

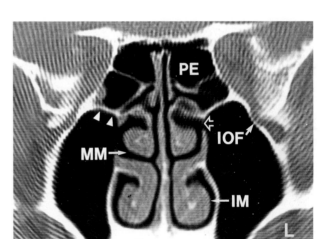

6.20

Figure **6.17**

Nasal septal spur. Note, in this CT scan, the massive nasal septal spur which is impinging onto the lateral nasal wall in the middle meatus (arrow).

Figure **6.18**

CT of an aerated nasal septum. This posterior portion of the perpendicular plate of the ethmoid is aerated (arrow).

Figure **6.19**

Normal maxillary sinus. THis CT scan demonstrates the anterior portion of the maxillary sinus (MS) draining through the maxillary ostia into the ethmoid infundibulum (open arrow). The infundibulum channel is bounded superolaterally by the ethmoid bulla (EB) and inferomedially by the uncinate process (UP). The ethmoid infundibulum opens into the semilunar hiatus. The semilunar hiatus is a two-dimensional, slit-like opening that connects the infundibulum to the middle meatus (short white arrow). The infraorbital foramen (IOF), inferior turbinate (IT) and inferior meatus (IM) are also shown.

Figure **6.20**

Accessory maxillary ostia. This coronal CT scan of the posterior ethmoid air cells (PE) and maxillary sinus demonstrates a large accessory maxillary sinus ostium on the right just lateral to the middle turbinate and a smaller one on left (open arrow) close to the posterior part of the middle meatus (MM). The thin plate of bone separating the superomedial margin of the maxillary sinus from the posterior ethmoid air cells is the ethmomaxillary plate (arrowheads). Note the inferior orbital fissure (IOF) and the inferior meatus (IM).

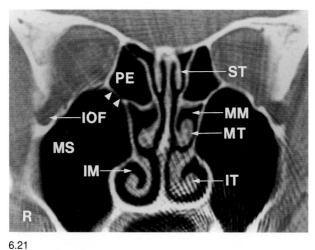

6.21

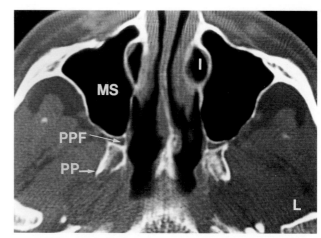

6.22

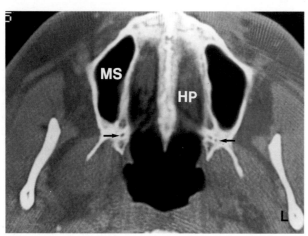

6.23

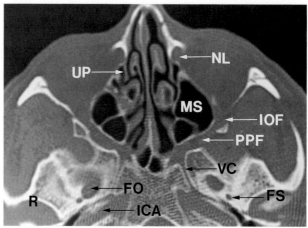

6.24

Figure **6.21**

The turbinates. This is a coronal CT scan through the middle portion of a normal maxillary sinus (MS). The superior (ST), middle (MT) and inferior (IT) turbinates with their corresponding superior, middle (MM), and inferior (IM) meatii, are clearly shown. The posterior ethmoid sinus (PE) is separated from the maxillary sinus by the ethmomaxillary plate (arrowheads).

Figure **6.22**

This normal axial CT scan demonstrates the maxillary sinus (MS), the pterygopalatine fossa (PPF) and the pterygoid process (PP). The superior aspect of the inferior meatus (I), is transected in this view.

Figure **6.23**

This normal axial CT scan demonstrates a section through the hard palate (HP), and the alveolar recesses of the maxillary sinuses (MS). The palatine foramina which transmit the greater and lesser palatine nerves are also shown (arrows).

Figure **6.24**

This normal axial CT scan demonstrates the uncinate process (UP) arising close to the wall of the nasolacrimal duct (NL). Also demonstrated are the pterygoid (vidian) canal (VC), the foramen ovale (FO), the foramen spinosum (FS) the pterygopalatine fossa (PPF), the infraorbital fissure (IOF), the maxillary sinus (MS) and the internal carotid artery (ICA).

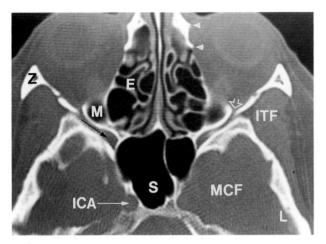

6.25

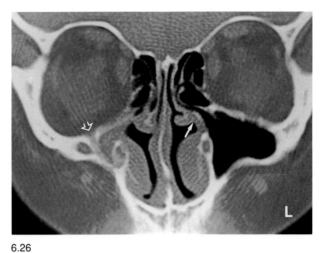

6.26

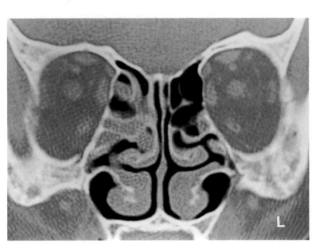

6.27

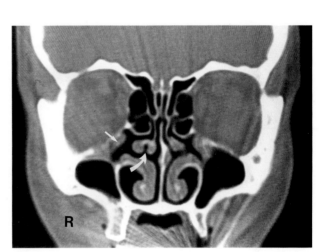

6.28

Figure **6.25**

This normal axial CT scan demonstrates the anterior and posterior lacrimal crests (arrowheads), the ethmoid labyrinth (E), the superior recess of the maxillary sinus (M), the zygoma (Z), the pterygopalatine fossa (black arrow), the inferior orbital foramen (open arrow), the infratemporal fossa (ITF), the middle cranial fossa (MCF), the sphenoid sinus (S) and the internal carotid artery (ICA).

Figure **6.27**

Hypoplasia of the maxillary sinus. This coronal CT scan demonstrates bilateral hypoplasia of the maxillary sinuses; consequently, the nasal cavity is wide and the floor of the orbit depressed.

Figure **6.26**

Hypoplasia of the maxillary sinus. This coronal CT scan demonstrates a hypoplastic maxillary sinus. Note that the right orbital floor lies at a lower level than the left orbital floor, with the right orbit showing apparent enlargement. The infraorbital nerve canal (open arrow) appears more laterally placed. On the left is a paradoxically bent middle turbinate that is apposed to the uncinate process (arrow).

Figure **6.28**

Hypoplasia of the maxillary sinus. On this CT the right maxillary sinus is atelectatic. Note how the posterior fontanelle has been laterally retracted. The uncinate process appears absent, but on closer inspection it can be seen adherent to the inferior orbital wall (arrow). An incidental finding is the sagittal groove which can be seen in the right middle turbinate (curved arrow).

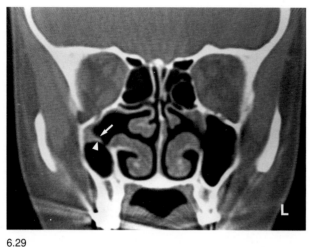

6.29

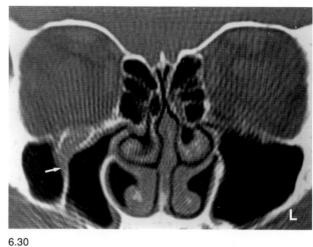

6.30

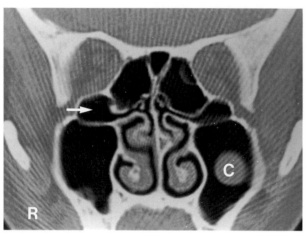

6.31

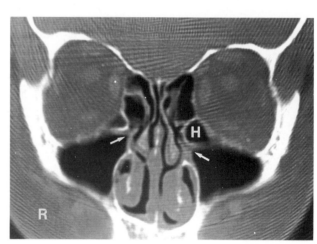

6.32

Figure **6.29**

Hypoplasia of the maxillary sinus. This is a more posterior CT scan of the patient in Figure 6.28. The 'fibrous septum' that is seen in the maxillary sinus (arrowhead) actually represents an invagination of the posterior fontanelle. The middle meatus is deep, as a result of lateral retraction of the large posterior fontanelle (arrow) into the maxillary sinus.

Figure **6.31**

CT of the ethmomaxillary sinus. Note the ethmomaxillary sinus (arrow) which is connected to the superior meatus by a short and medially directed bony channel. A small cyst (C) can be seen in the left maxillary sinus.

Figure **6.30**

Septated maxillary sinus. On this CT scan, a bony septum (arrow) is seen arising from the region of the infraorbital canal, which extends to the lateral wall dividing the right maxillary sinus into two unequal parts. These compartments usually communicate with each other through a defect somewhere in the septum.

Figure **6.32**

Haller's cells. On this CT scan, bilateral Haller's cells (H) compromising the ethmoid infundibulum on both sides are seen. Note the appositional changes (arrows) in the mucosa.

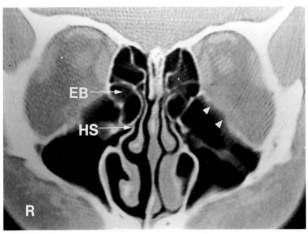

6.33

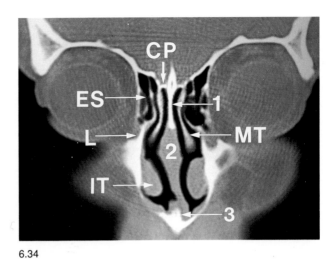

6.34

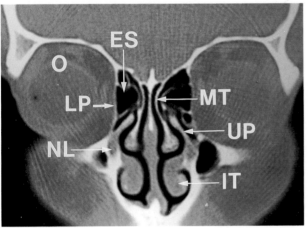

6.35

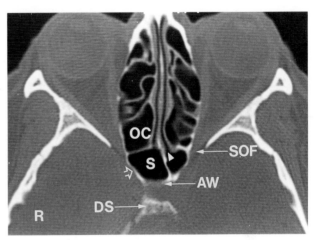

6.36

Figure **6.33**

Extensive Haller's cells. This CT scan demonstrates pneumatization of the floor of the left orbit from a posterolateral extension of a large Haller's cell. The floor of the orbit is thin and appears to be dehiscent (arrowheads). A large ethmoid bulla (EB) is seen on the right compromising the hiatus semilumaris (HS).

Figure **6.34**

CT of the anterior ethmoid sinuses and the nasal septum. The nasal septum is formed by the perpendicular plate of the ethmoid bone (1), the cartilaginous septum (2) and the vomer inferiorly (3). The anterior ethmoid cells (ES) are located lateral to the vertical insertion of the middle turbinate (MT). Note the lacrimal fossa (L), which contains the lacrimal sac, the cribriform plate (CP) and the anterior end of the inferior turbinate (IT).

Figure **6.35**

The anterior ethmoid sinuses. This is a more posterior CT scan than Figure 6.34. The lamina papyracea (LP) separates the anterior ethmoid cells (ES) from the orbit (O). The nasolacrimal duct (NL), the uncinate process (UP), inferior turbinate (IT) and the vertical insertion of the middle turbinate (MT) are also demonstrated in this anterior coronal scan.

Figure **6.36**

This normal axial CT scan demonstrates the posterior ethmoid Onodi's cell (OC), the superior orbital fissure (SOF), the sphenoid sinus (S), the sphenoid sinus ostium (arrowhead), the impression of the internal carotid artery (open arrow), and the anterior wall (AW) and posterior bone (DS) of the dorsum sella.

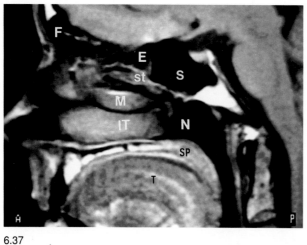

6.37

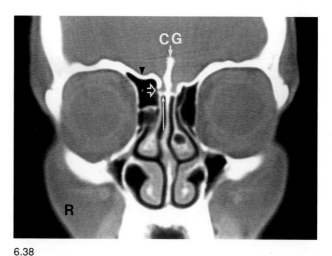

6.38

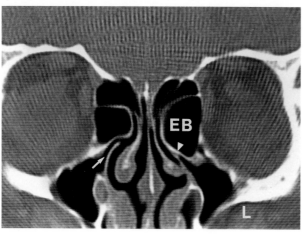

6.39

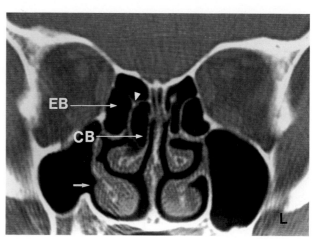

6.40

Figure **6.37**

Normal sagittal MR scan. This T1-weighted scan demonstrates the frontal sinus (F), the ethmoid sinus (E), the sphenoid sinus (S), the superior (st), the middle (M), and the inferior (IT) turbinates, as well as the nasopharynx (N), the soft palate (SP) and the tongue (T). Note that the posterior ethmoid cells are larger than the anterior cells.

Figure **6.38**

The cribriform plate and ethmoid fovea. The ethmoid fovea can clearly be seen to be both higher (arrowhead) and thicker than the cribriform plate (arrow) on this CT. This demonstrates the hazards of surgery in this area. Note the bony channel for the anterior ethmoidal artery on the right (open arrow). The crista galli is also demonstrated (CG). Other findings include bilateral bony hypertrophy of the middle turbinates and a small air cell in the left middle turbinate (concha bullosa).

Figure **6.39**

Large ethmoid bulla. On this CT scan, a large ethmoid bulla (EB) is present on the left side, obstructing the semilunar hiatus (arrowhead). The ethmoid infundibulum, semilunar hiatus and middle meatus on the right are normal (arrow).

Figure **6.40**

Large ethmoid bulla and concha bullosa. This patient presented with headaches. The coronal CT scan demonstrates a large ethmoid bulla (EB) in contact (arrowhead) with a large air cell in the vertical plate of the right middle turbinate (CB; a concha bullosa) on the right side. The patient had previously undergone a right intranasal antrostomy (arrow), but had remained symptomatic. Following resection of the ethmoid bulla and the middle turbinate air cell, the contact headaches were relieved.

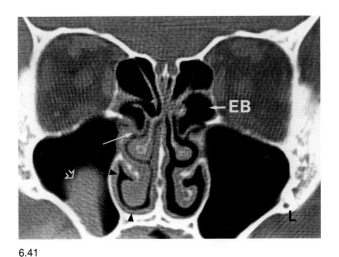

6.41

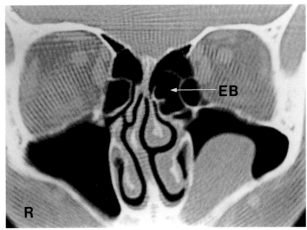

6.42

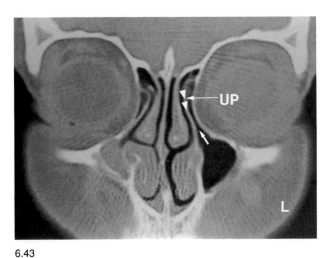

6.43

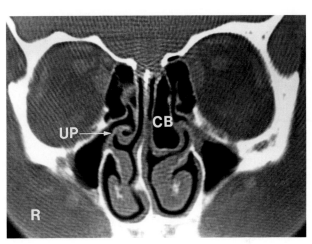

6.44

Figure **6.41**

Inferiorly extending ethmoid bullae. This coronal CT scan through the ostiomeatal complex demonstrates large ethmoid bullae (EB) overhanging the semilunar hiatus (arrow) with compromise of the ethmoid infundibulum and therefore the ventilation and drainage of the maxillary sinus. There is retained mucus (open arrow) in the floor of the maxillary sinus. Mucosal thickening can be seen in the inferior meatus and in the floor of the nasal cavity (arrowheads).

Figure **6.42**

Multiseptate ethmoid bulla. This CT scan demonstrates an enlarged left ethmoid bulla (EB) divided by multiple septae. The grossly enlarged bulla has compromised the frontal recess and the semilunar hiatus. There is a considerable amount of retained secretions in the left maxillary sinus; there is hypoplasia of the right maxillary sinus.

Figure **6.43**

The uncinate process. This coronal CT scan demonstrates the uncinate process (UP) inserting high into the lamina papyracea. The frontal recess (arrowheads) drains medial to the ethmoid infundibulum (arrow).

Figure **6.44**

Medially bent uncinate process. On this CT scan, the right uncinate process (UP) is seen to be turned medially and has come into intimate contact with the middle turbinate. Although the semilunar hiatus is not obstructed, the medially bent uncinate process is occluding the middle meatus. This scan also demonstrates a very large left-sided concha bullosa (CB), onto which the left uncinate process abuts.

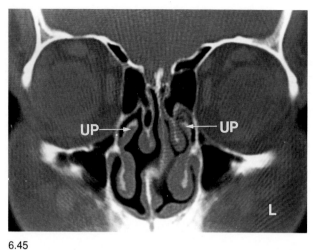

6.45

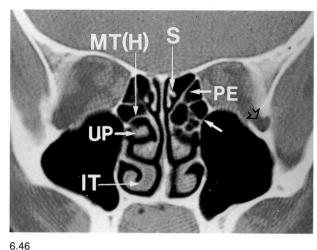

6.46

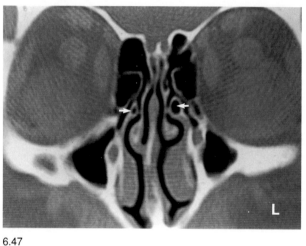

6.47

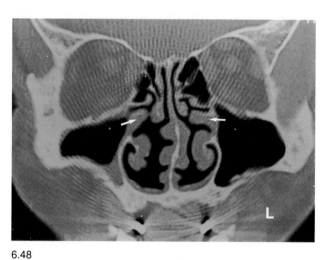

6.48

Figure **6.45**

Enlarge uncinate process. This CT scan shows grossly enlarged uncinate processes projecting anterior medially into the middle meatus (UP). On the left side, the middle meatus appears to be almost filled by the uncinate process. The nasal septum, which is deviated to the left side, shows evidence of previous trauma.

Figure **6.46**

Medially bent uncinate process. The right uncinate process (UP) in this coronal CT scan is medially bent to such an extent that it projects into the middle meatus. Note the inferior turbinate (IT) and the horizontal plate of the middle turbinates (MT(H)). The superior and the supreme turbinates (S). The ethmomaxillary plate (arrow), separates the maxillary sinus from the posterior ethmoid air cells (PE). The inferior orbital fissure is shown (open arrow).

Figure **6.47**

Pneumatized uncinate process. On this CT scan, both uncinate processes are pneumatized (arrows). The aerated uncinate process on the left is compromising the frontal recess and ethmoid infundibulum.

Figure **6.48**

Enlarged uncinate processes. This coronal CT scan demonstrates bilateral enlargement and medial deviation of the uncinate processes (arrows). These enlarged uncinate processes have narrowed the infundibula.

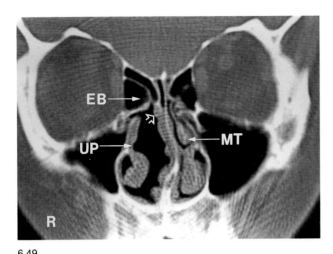

6.49

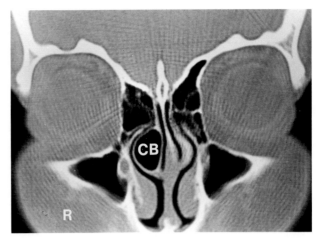

6.50

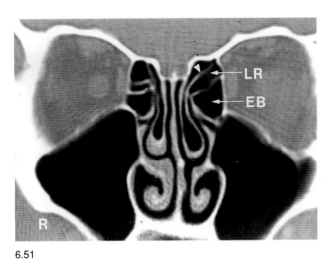

6.51

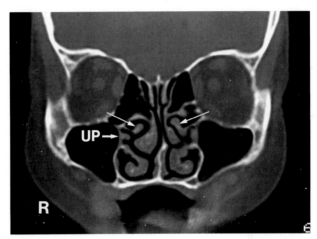

6.52

Figure **6.49**

Enlarged uncinate process. This patient presented with a history of nasal obstruction and recurrent sinusitis. There was no history of previous surgery; however, on the CT scan, the right middle turbinate was found to be vestigial (open arrow) and the uncinate process (UP) grossly enlarged. The right ethmoid bulla (EB) and the left middle turbinate (MT) are normal.

Figure **6.50**

Compromised ethmoid infundibulum. This large right-sided concha bullosa (CB) has reduced the adjacent infundibulum complex to a narrow slit. A paradoxical middle turbinate can be seen on the left.

Figure **6.51**

The lateral sinus. This coronal CT scan demonstrates bilateral concha bullosa. The horizontal insertion of the left middle turbinate (arrowhead) is seen. The space between the posterior margin of the ethmoid bulla (EB) and the horizontal insertion of the middle turbinate is the lateral recess (LR).

Figure **6.52**

Secondary middle turbinate. A secondary middle turbinate (arrows) is seen in both middle meatii on this CT scan. This anomaly should not be mistaken for a polyp. The uncinate process (UP) is bent medially in its posterior part.

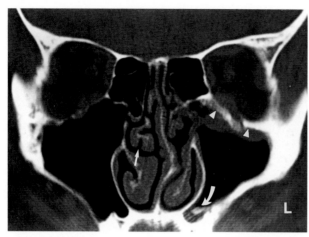

6.53

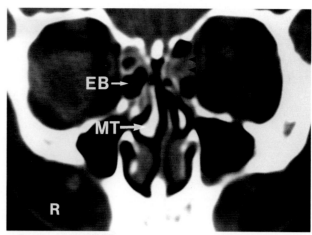

6.54

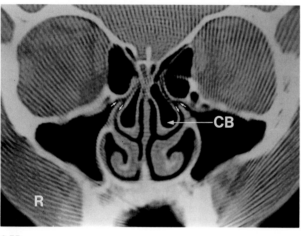

6.55

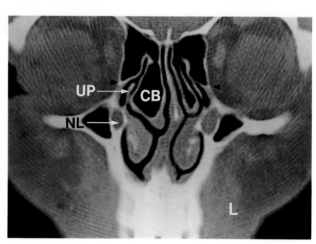

6.56

Figure **6.53**

Grooved middle turbinate. This CT scan demonstrates a sagittal groove (arrow) along the inferior free margin of the right middle turbinate. There is evidence of chronic sinusitis with reactive osteitis near the infraorbital canal (arrowheads), which is characteristic of benign disease. There is an unerupted tooth in the floor of the maxillary sinus (curved arrow).

Figure **6.54**

Bony hypertrophy of the middle turbinates: CT scan. Both wide- and soft-tissue window settings demonstrate that the right middle turbinate (MT) is predominantly bony with no soft tissue hypertrophy. This informs the surgeon that resection of this portion of the middle turbinate may be difficult. Inflammatory disease is seen in the right ethmoid infundibulum and in the left suprabullar space (black arrowheads). The ethmoid bulla (EB), is demonstrated.

Figure **6.55**

Concha bullosa. This CT scan demonstrates bilateral large concha bullosa (CB) with attendant narrowing of the ostiomeatal complexes and turbinate sinuses (small arrows).

Figure **6.56**

Bilateral concha bullosa (CB): CT scan. Note the pneumatization of the middle turbinates is derived from the ethmoid bulla. The ground lamella is seen to insert onto the lamina papyracea (arrowheads). The base of the uncinate processes (UP) inserts close to the nasolacrimal duct (NL).

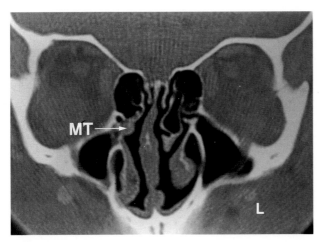

6.57

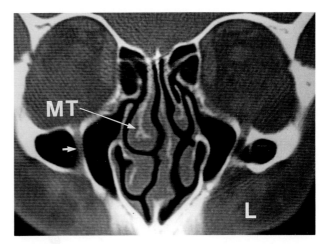

6.58

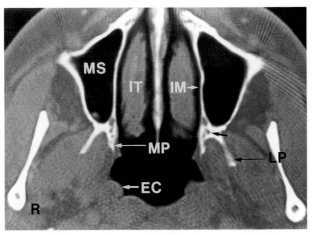

6.59

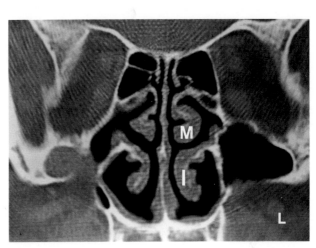

6.60

Figure **6.57**

Lateralized middle turbinate. Although small, this lateralized right middle turbinate (MT) is seen on the CT scan to be occluding the ostiomeatal complex. A left concha bullosa with aeration of the vertical plate is also seen.

Figure **6.58**

Soft-tissue hypertrophy of the middle turbinate. This CT scan demonstrates soft tissue hypertrophy of the right middle turbinate (MT). Despite this hypertrophy there is no evidence of compromise of the ostiomeatal complex. A slight deviation of the nasal septum to the left is apparent. The site of the infraorbital nerve is demonstrated (arrow).

Figure **6.59**

This normal axial CT scan demonstrates the maxillary sinuses (MS), the inferior turbinate (IT) and the inferior meatus (IM). Posterior to the maxillary sinus lies the medial (MP), and lateral pterygoid (LP), plates which enclose the pterygoid fossa. The palatine canals are shown (arrow). The eustachian cushion (EC), is shown protruding into the nasopharynx.

Figure **6.60**

Decongested inferior turbinates. This coronal CT scan shows the inferior turbinates to be small within a roomy nasal cavity. This is the characteristic appearance of the inferior turbinate following chronic use of topical decongestants. The thickened mucosa in the small right sided maxillary sinus follows from a previous Caldwell–Luc procedure. Normal inferior (I) and middle meati (M) are seen.

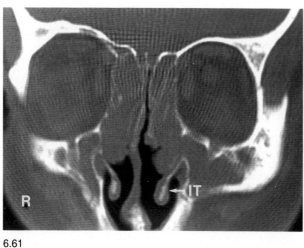

6.61

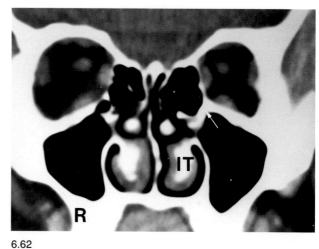

6.62

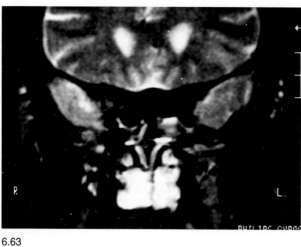

6.63

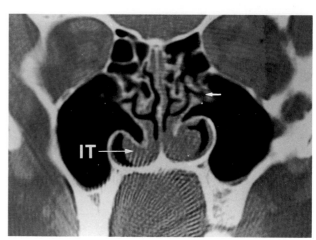

6.64

Figure **6.61**

Decongested inferior turbinates. This coronal CT scan demonstrates extensive polypoidal soft-tissue densities in the maxillary and ethmoid sinuses. As a consequence of the chronic abuse of topical decongestants the inferior turbinates (IT) are small and shrunken. There has been little effect on the middle turbinates. This is probably due to erectile tissue which is abundant on the inferior turbinate but which is limited in its distribution on the middle turbinate.

Figure **6.62**

Bony hypertrophy of the inferior turbinates. The narrow window scan demonstrates bony hypertrophy of the inferior turbinates (IT). The uncinate process is deviated medially leading to disease in the ethmoid infundibum (arrow). The orbital apex is also well demonstrated.

Figure **6.63**

Inferior turbinate hypertrophy. This patient has such extensive soft-tissue hypertrophy of the posterior ends of the inferior turbinates that the choanae are almost totally occluded. The turbinates are hyperintense in the T2-weighted MR scan.

Figure **6.64**

Pneumatized inferior turbinate: CT scan. The inferior turbinate is an independent bone articulating with a ridge on the medial aspect of the maxilla. Rarely, the inferior turbinate is incorporated into the maxilla and pneumatization of the inferior turbinate (IT) from the adjacent maxillary sinus may occur.

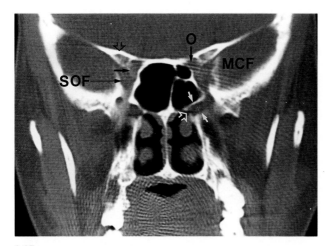

6.65

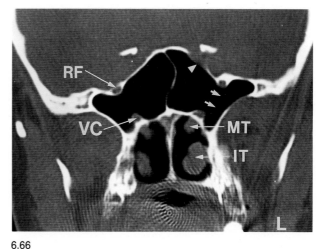

6.66

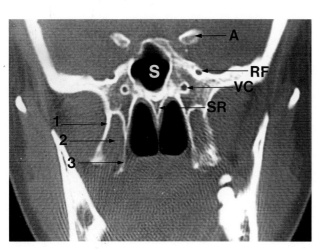

6.67

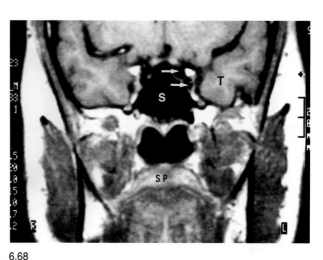

6.68

Figure **6.65**

The sphenoid sinus: CT scan. The sphenoethmoid recess (open white arrow) communicates with the pterygopalatine fossa through the sphenopalatine foramen (between white arrows). The optic foramen (O), is separated from the superior orbital fissure (SOF) by the optic strut (black arrow). The planum sphenoidale of the lesser wing of the sphenoid is demonstrated (open black arrow); the middle cranial fossa (MCF) is also seen.

Figure **6.66**

The sphenoid sinus: CT scan. The lateral recesses of the sphenoid sinus (arrows) and dehiscence of the roof of the sphenoid close to the optic nerve on the left side (arrowhead) can be seen, as well as the foramen rotundum (RF), pterygoid (vidian) canal (VC), and the posterior ends of the inferior turbinate (IT) and of the middle turbinate (MT).

Figure **6.67**

The sphenoid sinus. This CT scan demonstrates the sphenoid sinus (S), the foramen rotundum (RF), the pterygoid (vidian) canal (VC), the anterior clinoid process (A), the sphenoid rostrum (SR), as well as the lateral (1) and medial (2) pterygoid plates and the pterygoid fossa (3).

Figure **6.68**

The sphenoid sinus. This T1-weighted MR scan demonstrates the sphenoid sinus (S) and internal carotid artery (arrows) located on the lateral wall of the sinus. The other normal structures shown include the soft palate (SP) and the temporal lobes (T) in the middle cranial fossa.

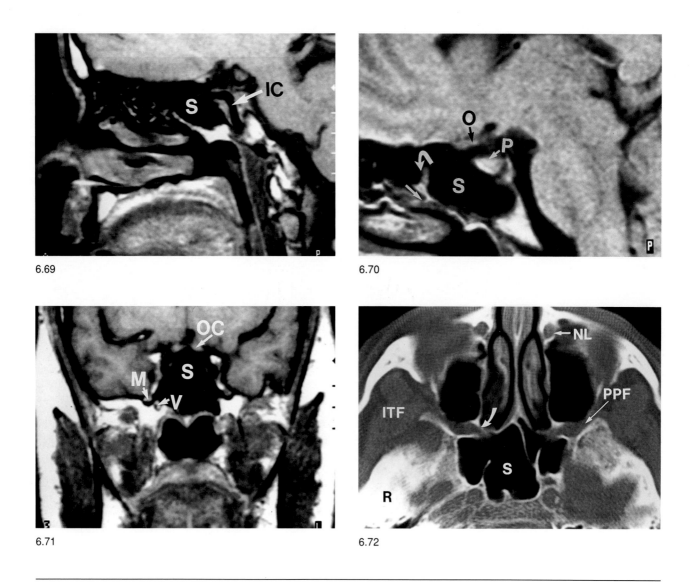

6.69

6.70

6.71

6.72

Figure **6.69**

The sphenoid sinus. This sagittal T1-weighted MR scan demonstrates the signal void internal carotid artery (IC), which is located close to the roof of the sinus (S).

Figure **6.70**

The sphenoid sinus. This sagittal T1-weighted MR scan demonstrates the normal sphenoid sinus (S) draining through an anterior placed opening close to the roof of the nasal vault (curved arrow). The small space (straight arrow) above the superior turbinate is the sphenoethmoid recess. The optic nerve (O) lies above and lateral to the sphenoid sinus and the pituitary gland (P) lies above the sinus.

Figure **6.71**

The sphenoid sinus. This coronal T1-weighted MR scan demonstrates the sphenoid sinus (S), the maxillary division of the trigeminal nerve running through the foramen rotundum (M), the vidian nerve within the pterygoid (vidian) canal (V) and the optic chiasm (OC).

Figure **6.72**

This normal axial CT scan demonstrates the nasolacrimal duct (NL), the sphenopalatine foramen (curved arrow), entering the pterygopalatine fossa (PPF), the sphenoid sinus (S), and the infratemporal fossa (ITF).

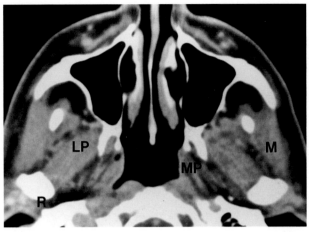

6.73

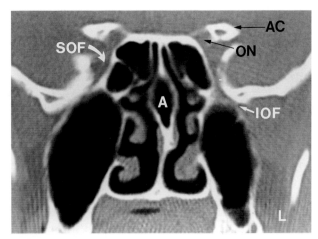

6.74

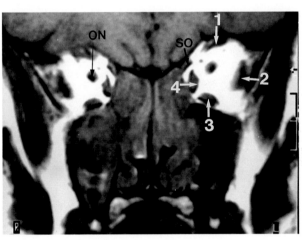

6.75

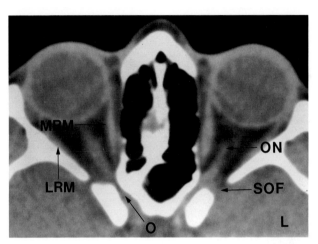

6.76

Figure **6.73**

This normal, narrow-window, axial CT scan demonstrates the muscles of mastication, namely the lateral pterygoid (LP), the medial pterygoid (MP), and masseter (M). The muscles are clearly separated by fat planes.

Figure **6.74**

Orbital apex. This CT scan demonstrates the normal characteristics of the inferior orbital fissure (IOF), the superior orbital fissure (SOF), the optic nerve (ON) and the anterior clinoids (AC). The nasal septum is pneumatized (A).

Figure **6.75**

The orbital apex. The orbital apex is well demonstrated on this coronal T1-weighted MR scan showing the medial rectus (4), lateral rectus (2), inferior rectus (3), superior rectus (1) and superior oblique (SO) muscles as well as the optic nerve (ON). This scan also demonstrates inflammatory and polypoidal disease in the sinuses. The fat in the orbit is bright on this T1-weighted sequence.

Figure **6.76**

The orbital apex and extraocular muscles. This axial CT scan demonstrates the bony optic canal (O), the optic nerve (ON) passing through this canal and the laterally placed superior orbital fissure (SOF). The medial (MRM) and lateral (LRM) rectus muscles are well demonstrated.

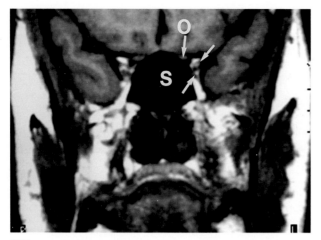

6.77

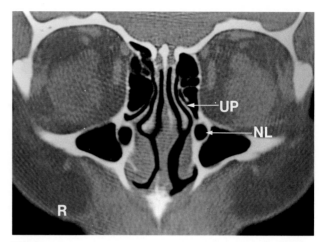

6.78

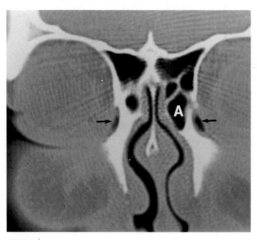

6.79

Figure **6.77**

The tendinous ring of Zinn (annulus of Zinn). This posterior coronal T1-weighted MR scan through the sphenoid sinus (S) demonstrates the tendinous ring of Zinn at the orbital apex, which gives origin to the recti muscles (arrows). The optic nerve (O) is superomedial to the annulus.

Figure **6.79**

Air in the lacrimal sac. The small air collections seen on this CT scan along the inferomedial aspect of the orbits are air within the lacrimal sac (arrows). This should not be mistaken for orbital emphysema following fracture or infection. An agger nasi cell is also demonstrated (A).

Figure **6.78**

The nasolacrimal duct. This anterior coronal CT scan demonstrates air in both nasolacrimal ducts (NL). The nasolacrimal duct is bounded by the maxilla, the lacrimal bone and the inferior turbinate. Both uncinate processes (UP) are elongated. Note the intimate relationship between the origin of the uncinate processes and the nasolacrimal duct.

7

The role of anatomic variants of the ostiomeatal complex and paranasal sinuses

As Messerklinger has stated, the ventilation and drainage of the anterior ethmoidal sinus, the maxillary sinus and the frontal sinus are dependent upon the convoluted clefts of the 'ostiomeatal complex' through which healthy, ciliated mucosa promotes optimal sinus ventilation and drainage. Most sinus infections are rhinogenic in origin and spread from the ostiomeatal complex to secondarily involve the frontal and the maxillary sinuses. The small clefts of the ostiomeatal complex in the lateral nasal wall are easily compromised or occluded by mucosal edema resulting in poor ventilation, failure of mucociliary clearance and stagnation of mucus and pus in the sinuses. This process is usually reversible; once the normal drainage pathways are reopened, the secondary disease within the larger maxillary and frontal sinuses usually resolves spontaneously. However, if there is an anatomic variant that narrows these key ethmoidal clefts, then minimal mucosal edema will predispose the patient to recurrent infections and may result in chronic inflammatory changes in the mucosa.

Previously, surgical procedures to alleviate recurrent or chronic inflammatory episodes have been directed at the larger paranasal sinuses. The ventilation of these sinuses was improved by creating new and theoretically effective alternative drainage pathways and by resecting a large amount of bone and diseased mucosa. Additional drainage procedures, such as inferior meatal antrostomies, are now known not to redirect the mucosal flow through the newly created opening but only to act as a drain when the mucociliary system is overwhelmed by mucus and pus. The persistence of symptoms following these procedures is usually secondary to disease in the anterior ethmoid, affecting the natural ostia and the ostiomeatal complex. Recurrent sinus infections may also occur despite there being a widely patent natural accessory ostium when ostiomeatal complex disease is present (Figure 7.1 and 7.2).

Functional endoscopic sinus surgery is directed at the natural drainage pathways. The limited surgical resection of tissue, to widen the natural clefts and improve sinus ventilation, has led to the reversal of mucosal disease in the larger paranasal sinuses. The direct endoscopic visualization of the small clefts of the ostiomeatal complex is limited, but computed tomography (CT), especially in the coronal plane, is complementary in defining the anatomy, and the site and extent of disease in the paranasal sinuses and in the surrounding soft tissues.

Those anatomic variants that may compromise the ostiomeatal complex and promote recurrent sinusitis are discussed in this chapter and in chapter 6.

The various structures that are adjacent to the drainage pathway of the major sinuses can compromise the drainage if these structures are large or deflected from their normal position. The important variations are listed in Table 7.1.

AGGER NASI CELLS

The extent of pneumatization of the agger mound can be clearly seen on CTs in the coronal plane. Agger nasi cells are usually pneumatized from the frontal recess. Enlarged agger nasi cells may involve the frontal recess either mechanically by obstructing the recess, if they are well developed, or by the direct spread of inflammation. Inflammation may also spread through a dehiscence of the lateral nasal wall to involve the orbit or the lacrimal sac (Figure 7.3; see also Figure 6.13).

AERATED CRISTA GALLI

A pneumatized crista galli may become involved by benign inflammatory disease and present clinically

---

Table **7.1**   Important anatomic structures of the ostiomeatal complex and their variations.

Structure	Variation
Ethmoid bulla	Enlarged, obstructing the ethmoid infundibulum, semilunar hiatus and/or middle meatus
Middle turbinate	Hypertrophy Concha bullosa Paradoxically bent middle turbinate
Uncinate process	Medially or laterally deflected Pneumatization Hypertrophy
Haller's cell	When present and enlarged, can obstruct the natural ostium of the maxillary sinua and the infundibulum
Nasal septum	Deviation of the nasal septum and septal spurs
Agger nasi cells	When present and enlarged, can obstruct the frontal recess

---

with headaches. Clinical examination and plain radiographs are normal in the majority of these cases; however, CT in the coronal plane will demonstrate the air cell within the crista galli. This air cell usually drains into the frontal recess, and both of these regions are usually involved simultaneously with inflammatory disease (Figure 7.3 and 7.4). If the ostium of this air cell is occluded, a mucocele of the crista galli may develop.

UNCINATE PROCESS

The uncinate process has an intimate relationship with the ethmoid infundibulum and the middle meatus. The commonest anatomic variant associated with inflammatory disease of the adjacent paranasal sinuses is a medial deviation of the uncinate process. The uncinate process may abut the middle turbinate, thus obstructing the middle meatus (Figures 7.5 and 7.6).

A long or a thickened uncinate process will narrow the semilunar hiatus between its posterior margin and the ethmoid bulla, especially if the bulla is well pneumatized (Figure 7.7).

A swollen, inflamed uncinate process is clearly visualized by endoscopy, but pneumatization of the uncinate process cannot be differentiated from hypertrophy by endoscopy (see Figure 6.49).

THE FRONTAL RECESS

Whether the frontal recess opens into the ethmoid infundibulum is determined by the superior insertion of the uncinate process, as discussed in Chapter 3. This superior insertion determines whether the frontal recess and frontal sinus are at risk from inflammation spreading from the anterior ethmoid and maxillary sinuses. If the uncinate process inserts laterally onto the lamina papyracea, this is less likely as the frontal recess in this situation drains directly into the middle meatus. If, however, the uncinate process inserts superiorly into the roof of the ethmoid or medially into the middle turbinate, then the frontal recess will drain into the ethmoid infundibulum.

The frontal recess may also be compromised by anatomic variations of the surrounding anatomic structures, such as well-developed agger nasi cells, a prominent ethmoid bulla, a concha bullosa or abnormalities of the uncinate process (Figure 7.8). Inflammatory disease within these structures (Figure 7.3) or in the lateral recess may spread into the frontal sinus and thus interfere with the ventilation and drainage of the frontal sinus (Figure 7.9).

CONCHA BULLOSA

Concha bullosa is the term used to refer to a pneumatized middle turbinate. When large, a concha bullosa may compromise the middle meatus and ostiomeatal complex (Figures 7.10 and 7.11). If a hypertrophied or pneumatized middle turbinate protrudes anteriorly, it may obstruct the frontal recess (see Figures 6.66 and 6.68).

The air cell within a concha bullosa is lined with respiratory epithelium and thus is predisposed to the same inflammatory disorders that can occur in any paranasal sinus. An acute sinusitis or concha bullitis may be demonstrated as an air–fluid level (Figure 7.12), or bubbles of air may be seen within the retained secretions (Figures 7.8 and 7.13).

Occlusion of the ostium of a concha bullosa may result in the development of a mucocele, the clinical features of which are nasal obstruction and headaches (Figure 7.12). As with any other mucocele, secondary infection will result in a pyocele (Figure 7.14). Resection of the lateral plate of the middle turbinate is indicated.

CT is less helpful in diagnosing a concha bullosa in the presence of extensive sinonasal polyposis. In this situation, the normal demarcation planes of air, bone and soft tissue are obscured, and detail cannot always be ascertained (Figure 7.15).

ETHMOID BULLA

The ethmoid bulla may be the site of inflammatory disease or it may predispose the patient to inflammatory disease by obstructing the ostiomeatal complex. It is unusual to find isolated ethmoid bullitis (Figure 7.16), and the ethmoid bulla is more commonly involved in generalized inflammatory disease of the ethmoid sinus (Figure 7.17).

If the ethmoid bulla is large, it may obstruct the middle meatus by impinging on the middle turbinate and so cause headaches and nasal obstruction without any inflammatory changes in the adjacent paranasal sinuses (see Figure 6.38). However, the ethmoid bulla may also predispose to recurrent or chronic inflammation in the adjacent sinus if its configuration causes obstruction of the ostiomeatal complex (Figures 7.17 and 7.18). A large ethmoid bulla may overhang the semilunar hiatus (see Figure 6.35), or it may reduce the lumen of the ethmoid infundibulum, reducing the ventilation and drainage of the adjacent sinuses.

THE LATERAL SINUS

The lateral sinus is a variably present space. When present, the lateral sinus is located posterior to the ethmoid bulla and anterior to the ground lamella. It may extend above the ethmoid bulla, as the suprabullar space, and communicate anteriorly with the frontal recess. The lateral sinus normally drains into the posterosuperior aspect of the semilunar hiatus which is also called the superior recess of the semilunar hiatus. The lateral sinus may be obstructed by an enlarged ethmoid bulla, a concha bullosa, or an edematous or hypertrophic uncinate process (Figure 7.19). If the lateral sinus communicates with the frontal recess, then inflammatory disease may spread along this route (Figures 7.20 and 7.21).

HALLER'S CELLS

Haller's cells are thought to arise from the anterior ethmoid sinus and project in a variable manner into the inferomedial aspect of the orbital floor, opposite the natural ostium of the maxillary sinus. Haller's cells may be an incidental finding or, when enlarged, they may predispose to recurrent or chronic inflammatory disease in the maxillary and frontal sinuses by narrowing the ethmoid infundibulum (Figures 7.15 and 7.22).

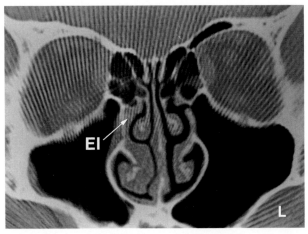

7.1

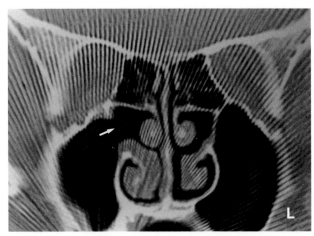

7.2

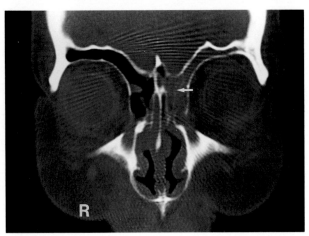

7.3

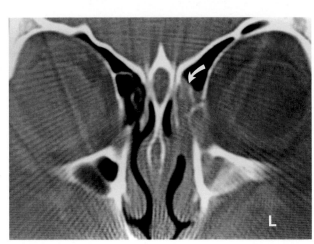

7.4

Figure **7.1**

Obstruction of the ethmoid infundibulum: CT scan. Disease in the right ethmoid infundibulum is seen occluding the natural ostia (EI).

Figure **7.2**

Accessory maxillary sinus ostium: CT scan. A large patent posterior fontanelle can be seen on the right (arrow). The ventilation and drainage of the maxillary sinus occurs primarily through the natural ostium even when there is an accessory ostium.

Figure **7.3**

Frontal recess disease: CT scan. The left frontal recess (arrow) is occluded by inflammatory disease.

Figure **7.4**

Pneumatized crista galli: CT scan. The pneumatized crista galli (curved arrow) is occluded by inflammatory disease.

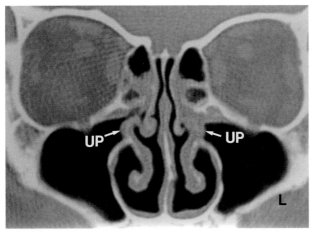

7.5

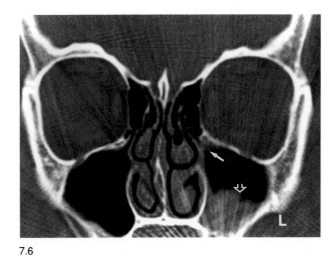

7.6

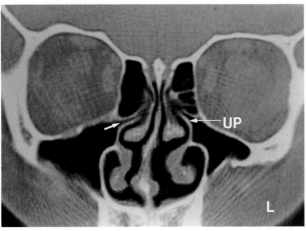

7.7

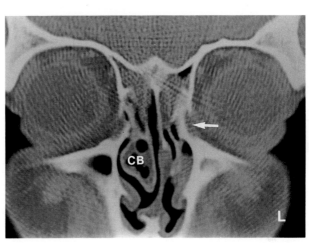

7.8

Figure **7.5**

Medially deviated uncinate process: CT scan. Medial deflection of the uncinate processes (UP) results in compromise of the middle meatus. As a result, inflammatory changes have occurred in the left ostiomeatal unit.

Figure **7.6**

Obstruction of the ethmoid infundibulum. The coronal CT scan demonstrates early compromise of the infundibulum caused by edema of the mucosa (arrow). As a result there is inflammatory debris in the floor of the maxillary sinus (open arrow). Surgery comprising of excision of the uncinate process and establishing an adequate middle meatal antrostomy would lead to resolution of the maxillary sinus disease.

Figure **7.7**

Uncinate process: CT scan. A long uncinate process (UP) can obstruct the semilunar hiatus, especially if the ethmoid bulla is large; the ethmoid infundibulum is arrowed.

Figure **7.8**

Inflammatory disease in a concha bullosa. This coronal CT scan demonstrates a large diseased concha bullosa (CB) extending far anteriorly compromising the premeatal region and the frontal recess. Inflammatory disease is seen in both frontal sinuses. Normally, the middle turbinate is not seen in the anterior coronal CT scans where the frontal sinus and the lacrimal fossa (arrow) are visualized.

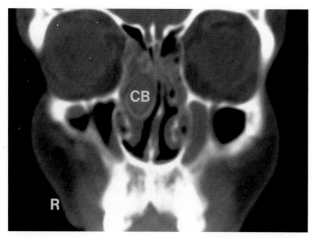

7.9

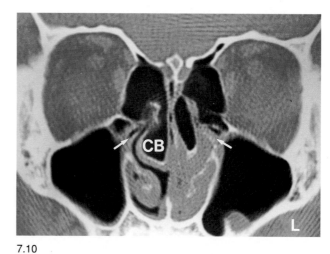

7.10

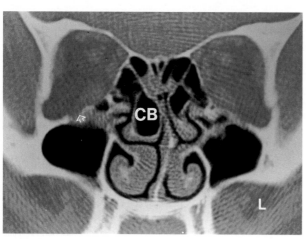

7.11

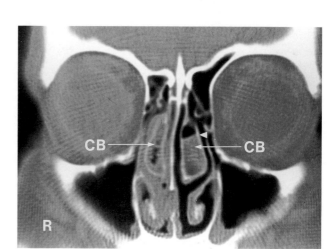

7.12

Figure **7.9**

Concha bullosa mucocele. This is a coronal CT scan of the patient shown in Figure 7.14. Note the huge mucus-filled concha bullosa (CB) which extends both inferiorly and laterally and compromises the middle meatus.

Figure **7.11**

Concha bullosa. This coronal CT scan demonstrates an unusual configuration of the middle turbinate (CB) with pneumatization of the horizontal portion of the middle turbinate. The floor of the orbit is thin (open arrow) close to the ethmoid infundibulum. This emphasizes the value of the preoperative scan so that inadvertent entrance into the orbits may be prevented.

Figure **7.10**

Bilateral concha bullosa: CT scan. The large air cell in the left middle turbinate (CB) has produced apposition of the middle and the inferior turbinates. The large ethmoid bulla together with the concha bullosa has occluded the left middle meatus; the ethmoid infundibulum is arrowed.

Figure **7.12**

Concha bullitis: CT scan. Note the air–fluid level in the left concha bullosa (arrowhead). There is inflammatory disease in the right concha bullosa (CB), with significant compromise of the adjacent ostiomeatal complex.

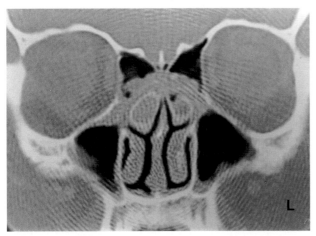

7.13

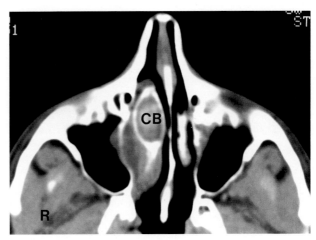

7.14

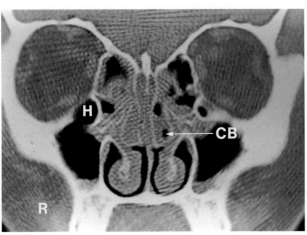

7.15

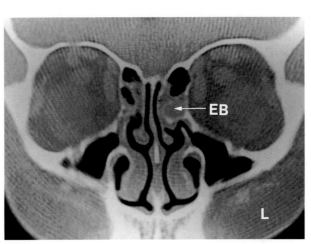

7.16

Figure **7.13**

Concha bullosa mucocele. Coronal CT scan demonstrates bilateral mucocele of the concha bullosa, with extensive ostiomeatal complex disease.

Figure **7.14**

Concha bullosa mucocele. This axial CT scan demonstrates a large mucocele of the coronal bullosa (CB) with mucosal enhancement. This patient would have remained symptomatic if surgery aimed specifically at the middle turbinate had not been undertaken.

Figure **7.15**

Ostiomeatal complex disease. This CT scan shows extensive ostiomeatal complex disease as well as disease in both conchae bullosa (CB). The narrowed ethmoid infundibulum are further compromised by Haller's cells (H).

Figure **7.16**

Enlarged ethmoid bulla: CT scan. The ethmoid bulla (EB) in this patient extends medially to such an extent that it has come into contact with the vertical plate of the middle turbinate. Note the isolated inflammatory disease seen within the lumen of this medially protruding ethmoid bulla.

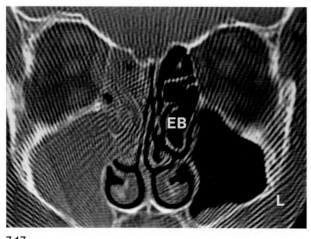

7.17

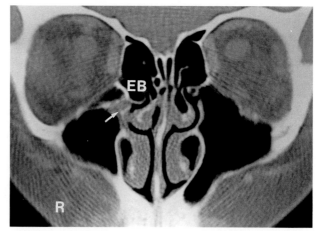

7.18

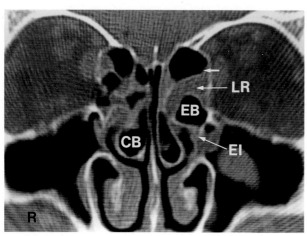

7.19

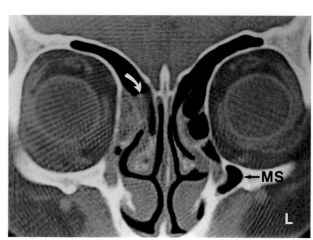

7.20

Figure **7.17**

Large ethmoid bulla. This CT scan demonstrates a large ethmoid bulla (EB) overhanging the semilunar hiatus on the left side. Similar findings on the right side resulted in a unilateral ethmomaxillary sinusitis.

Figure **7.18**

Large ethmoid bulla. This CT scan demonstrates early compromises of the right maxillary sinus ostia and ethmoid infundibulum (arrow), with a large ethmoid bulla (EB) overhanging the semilunar hiatus. This has resulted in early infundibular disease.

Figure **7.19**

Lateral sinus disease. This CT scan demonstrates a normal ethmoid bulla (EB), a concha bullosa (CB) and inflammatory disease in the lateral sinus (LR). The ground lamella (arrow) is shown as is the occluded ethmoid infundibulum (EI).

Figure **7.20**

Frontal recess draining into the lateral sinus: CT scan. The frontal recess (curved arrow) is occluded by inflammatory disease. There is also disease in the anterior ethmoid air cells. The anterior aspect of the maxillary sinus is shown (MS).

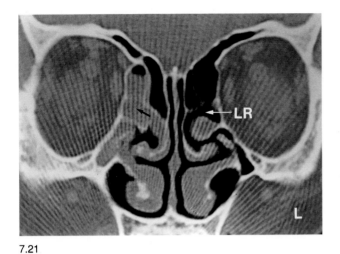

7.21

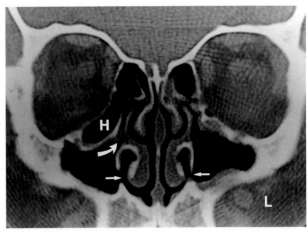

7.22

Figure **7.21**

Frontal recess draining into the lateral sinus. This CT scan demonstrates disease in the right lateral recess (arrow). The lateral sinus on the left (LR) is normal. The maxillary sinus is small and hypoplastic.

Figure **7.22**

Haller's cell: CT scan. This patient has a large Haller's cell on the right side (H). The right infundibulum is severely compromised by this huge Haller's cell (curved arrow). Despite previous drainage procedures (arrows), this patient presented with recurrent sinus disease.

8

The radiologic appearance of benign inflammatory paranasal sinus disease

ACUTE SINUSITIS

Acute sinusitis is characterized clinically by nasal obstruction, purulent nasal discharge, postnasal drip and facial pain. The characteristics and distribution of the pain or headache may help the clinician locate the origin of the disease. The pain of frontal sinusitis radiates to the forehead and is usually associated with a generalized headache. In acute maxillary sinusitis, the pain usually radiates from the inner canthus to the cheek. The pain may also radiate to the alveolar region, mimicking dental disease. Ethmoid sinusitis is associated with pain that tends to localize to the bridge of the nose and behind the medial canthus of the eye. It is often cyclical, being worse first thing in the morning after rising. Sphenoid sinusitis is now realized to be generally underdiagnosed. It usually occurs as part of a pansinusitis, but it may arise in isolation, leading to occipital or vertical headache as well as retro-orbital pain. In all types of sinusitis the pain is more severe if the ostium of the sinus becomes totally obstructed and an empyema forms. This situation is dangerous clinically, because lytic lesions may develop in the sinus walls leading to intraorbital or intracranial sepsis.

Plain radiographs are usually adequate for the investigation of patients with symptoms suggestive of an uncomplicated acute sinusitis (Figure 8.1). Plain radiographs are also useful for the documentation of sinus infections in the frontal, maxillary or sphenoid sinuses. A Water's view is usually sufficient for follow up examination of those patients with sinusitis of these larger paranasal sinuses. The mucosa will be thickened and, if mucus or pus collects in the sinus, an air–fluid interface will be evident (Figure 8.1). If the radiologist is uncertain about the existence of an air–fluid level, the patient's head can be tilted to one side by 45° and the radiograph repeated. In severe sinusitis, the extensive mucosal edema and fluid

exudate will make the sinus appear totally opaque. The infection may be confined to only one cavity (usually the maxillary or the frontal sinus), or it may involve all of the sinuses on one side as a pansinusitis. Spread of infection from the anterior ethmoid complex to the posterior ethmoid sinus is usually through defects in the ground lamella. If an empyema develops, plain radiographs will not exhibit any changes other than that of an acute sinusitis, i.e. the bony walls of the sinus do not bow outwards and there is no expansion of the sinus lumen. On computed tomography (CT), however, rarefaction of the sinus walls may be seen in addition to the opacification of the sinus and will indicate that a major complication is imminent if the infection is not controlled. Recurrent infection suggests that the dental roots should be examined, as disease in the roots may be a predisposing factor.

Plain radiographs of an infected frontal sinus will reveal loss of definition of the superior bony margin, with mucosal thickening. Opacification may be minimal in the acute phase, becoming more marked with chronicity.

In patients who are immunocompromised, the symptoms and signs of acute sinusitis may be disproportionately insignificant to the danger they present. Clinical features of fever, rhinorrhea, sinus tenderness and facial edema may only give rise to radiologic evidence of mucosal thickening. This finding should not be disregarded as the patients are often unable to mount the appropriate inflammatory response, i.e. produce a purulent exudate in the sinus. Sinus infections in the immunocompromised patient can easily spread intracranially. Delayed diagnosis and treatment may result in fulminant infection which can be fatal. Opaque sinuses may indicate bony involvement, with or without destruction by the infection, and the outlook is poor (Figures 8.2 and 8.3).

CHRONIC SINUSITIS

The symptoms of chronic sinusitis are variable, sometimes being severe but more often being mild. There is usually a combination of nasal obstruction, rhinorrhea and postnasal drip. Epistaxis, anosmia or cacosmia and vestibulitis may also be associated with chronic sinusitis. Patients frequently present with recurrent headaches and facial pain.

The radiologic features of chronic sinusitis are similar to those of acute sinusitis if there is an acute process superimposed on the chronic disease. The mucoperiosteum becomes thickened, and chronic fibrosis with polypoid proliferation and retained secretions contribute to the opacification of the sinuses involved (Figures 8.4–8.6). Recurrent or chronic sinusitis will produce an osteitis with new bone formation along the contours of the sinus cavity. The extent of the osteitis is proportionate to the frequency of infection and the length of the history. The resulting sclerosis can lead to thickening of the sinus wall and a diminished volume of the sinus cavity (Figures 8.7–8.9). The sinus walls may be eroded by chronic benign inflammation, usually occurring along the medial wall of the maxillary sinus and around the infraorbital canal. If chronic infections occur during childhood, the sinus may remain small and hypoplastic.

FUNGAL INFECTIONS OF THE PARANASAL SINUSES

Fungal sinusitis is an unusual condition that is being recognized with increasing frequency. It is caused mainly by *Aspergillus*, but fungi of the Mucoraceae group are also implicated. The disease can present in two forms, either as extramucosal disease or as the more dangerous fulminant form. The extramucosal disease presents with symptoms that are not dissimilar to chronic sinusitis, with nasal obstruction, purulent rhinorrhea and facial pain, all of which are resistant to treatment with antibiotics (Figures 8.10 and 8.11). This may be associated with the slow development of a fungus ball. The fulminant form of fungal sinusitis usually occurs in immunosuppressed or uncontrolled diabetic patients with ketoacidosis and has, in the past, been primarily attributed to mucormycosis, especially as this occurs in the aggressive rhinocerebral form. Necrosis of the turbinates, with black crusting in the nasal cavity, is suggestive of this aggressive form of invasive fungal

sinusitis. However, *Aspergillus* is becoming increasingly discovered to be as dangerous in some clinical groups. Both *Aspergillus* and the Mucoraceae can cause vasculitis, mycotic aneurysms, and thrombosis and may spread intracranially causing hemorrhage and infarction (Figures 8.2 and 8.3). The diagnosis may be suspected from the clinical features and characteristic features identified on subsequent radiographs, and is confirmed by examination of nasal scrapings and mucosal biopsies.

The findings on plain radiographs and on conventional tomographs include nodular mucoperiosteal thickening, absent air–fluid levels, clouding of the ethmoid sinuses and bony erosion. There may also be areas of increased attenuation which represent calcium phosphate and calcium sulphate in the necrotic fungal mass (Figures 8.10 and 8.11). Sclerotic thickening of the bony walls of the sinusitis, with both remodeling and destruction, can be seen in some cases. It may be impossible to radiologically differentiate fungal sinusitis from malignancy, especially when there is extensive bony destruction.

Areas of increased attenuation in a diseased sinus, in the absence of intravenous contrast administration, are readily identified by CT and are highly suggestive of fungal infection. Heavy metals such as iron and magnesium are essential components of fungal metabolism. It is these heavy metals that cause the high-density signal on CT. The nodular mucoperiosteal thickening and bony sclerosis and erosion are clearly documented. The differential diagnosis of such a high-density area includes high-density polyps and inverting papilloma with dystrophic calcification.

Magnetic resonance imaging (MR) evaluation of this condition can be diagnostic. There is a decreased signal intensity in the T1- and T2-weighted MR sequences, due to the presence in the fungal concretions of iron, magnesium and manganese, which are known to be essential to the fungal amino-acid metabolism, and calcium. These metals are an essential ingredient for fungal amino-acid metabolism (see Chapter 12).

Fungal sinusitis is treated with a combination of systemic antifungal agents and surgical débridement.

COMPLICATIONS OF SINUSITIS

The complications of sinusitis are usually related to disease of the frontoethmoid complex, sphenoid

Table **8.1** Complications of sinusitis

Local	Orbital	Intracranial
Empyema	Preseptal cellulitis	Meningitis
Mucocele	Subperiosteal abscess	Epidural empyema or abscess
Pyocele	Intraorbital abscess	Brain abscess
Osteitis	Endophthalmitis	Cavernous sinus thrombosis
Osteomyelitis	Optic neuritis	Superior sagittal sinus thrombosis
Facial cellulitis	Superior orbital fissure syndrome	Multiple cranial nerve palsies from meningitis
	Occlusion of central retinal artery	

sinus and their adjacent structures. These complications are potentially life-threatening, and may be considered in three groups: local, orbital and intracranial. The various complications are listed in Table 8.1. In the pre-antibiotic era it was not uncommon to see osteomyelitis or intraorbital abscesses. With the widespread use of antibiotics there has been a significant decline in the incidence of such complications and they now more commonly occur in association with resistant bacteria or immunocompromised patients, such as those with AIDS. Very few patients with sinusitis develop intracranial or orbital sepsis. Congenital deficiencies of the sinus walls, fractures or surgical defects may predispose some individuals to such complications. The infection spreads through various portals, including along the interstitium surrounding the veins, through emissary foramina and through the diploic veins. Perineural spread may occur around the branches of the olfactory nerve traversing the cribriform plate.

These complications need immediate treatment with high-dose intravenous antibiotics and often require surgical drainage. If such treatment is instituted without delay, permanent ocular and neurologic damage may be avoided. Even though magnetic resonance imaging is of diagnostic value, the patients are usually too ill and too uncooperative to undergo this lengthier examination. Thus the diagnosis is often confirmed by CT, which is conducted in both the axial and the coronal planes following the administration of intravenous contrast. The scans should be examined with both wide- and narrow-window settings, to allow adequate assessment of the sinus cavities, the bony walls and the soft-tissue structures.

Osteomyelitis

Osteomyelitis affects the frontal bone most commonly, the maxillary sinus being the second most commonly affected. Osteomyelitis of the frontal bone is either spontaneous or occurs following trauma, either accidental or operative. The sepsis spreads directly or via thrombophlebitis of the diploic veins. Osteomyelitis occurs with infection of diploetic bone, and osteitis is due to infection of compact bone, such as is found in the floor of the frontal sinus. For this reason, surgical drainage of an acute frontal sinusitis should only be undertaken through the sinus floor.

Osteomyelitis tends to manifest itself as a subperiosteal abscess limited by the attachment of the periosteum or, intracranially, by the dura (an extradural abscess). Clinically, osteomyelitis of the frontal bone presents with a soft doughy swelling of the frontal bone. The patient is unwell, with a fever, rigors, diffuse headache and spreading edema of the forehead. This condition, with an extradural abscess, subperiosteal abscess and intervening osteomyelitis, is known as Pott's puffy tumor.

There may be little radiologic evidence for 7–10 days if the osteomyelitis is untreated. When radiologic change occurs there is poor definition of the sinus walls with the disruption of the mucoperiosteal lining. If the infection is not controlled at this stage with high-dose antibiotics, the bone becomes less dense and lytic lesions appear in the adjacent bone. The appearance on plain radiographs is similar to that on CT, with unevenly distributed multiple lytic foci (Figures 8.12–8.14). Bony sequestra are less common in chronic osteomyelitis of the facial bones or skull than in chronic osteomyelitis of the long bones. In chronic cases, sclerotic changes are superimposed over areas of rarefaction, and the margins of the sinus become indistinct. Following intravenous contrast administration the acutely inflamed mucosa exhibits intense enhancement. This should be differentiated from the enhancement of pyoceles. The smooth expansion of the sinus walls associated with pyoceles is usually absent with osteomyelitis.

Osteomyelitis following maxillary sinusitis usually affects the alveolar bone, which is cancellous, between two plates of thin compact bone. It may occur in both adults and in infants. The commonest cause is dental infection, and it may lead to a subperiosteal abscess spreading across the maxilla. Radiologic features are minimal in some cases with slight opacity of the maxillary sinus. In some cases there may be marked sclerosis of the maxilla.

Intraorbital complications

Intraorbital complications include cellulitis, subperiosteal abscess, orbital abscess, thrombosis of the superior and/or inferior ophthalmic veins, optic neuritis and central artery occlusion. These complications are usually associated with infection of the frontal or ethmoid sinuses or with a pansinusitis. The usual route of spread is either through bony dehiscences of the sinus wall or through the valveless venous pathways. The patient may become blind if treatment, such as high-dose intravenous antibiotics, abscess drainage and orbital decompression (if indicated), is not commenced immediately.

An important clinical differentiation must be made in this group regarding the position of the focus of infection in relation to the orbital septum, i.e. the fibrous band that spans from the orbital margins to the tarsal plates. Both preseptal and postseptal orbital inflammation present with swelling of the upper eyelid. The skin assumes a dusky, reddish blue hue. In a case of preseptal orbital cellulitis the eye will be found in its normal position, and will have normal movements if the lids are prised apart. Postseptal inflammation can be divided into two groups, each requiring different management. These infactions are either extraconal, i.e. subperiosteal, or they are intraconal, i.e. within the periosteum.

Extraconal orbital cellulitis is associated with exophthalmos of the globe, restricted eye movements and chemosis of the conjunctiva, and

vision may rapidly deteriorate. This condition requires aggressive treatment with intravenous antibiotics and surgical drainage of any abscess collection, using the same approach as used for an external ethmoidectomy. Orbital decompression may also be indicated. The commonest cause of extraconal inflammation is ethmoiditis.

Intraconal inflammation has similar clinical features, such as exophthalmos, restricted eye movements and chemosis, but there may also be papilledema of the optic disc and there is a grave risk of retrograde infection causing cavernous sinus thrombosis. If intraorbital abscess formation occurs there is usually marked exophthalmos and rapid decrease in the visual acuity. Again the treatment is aggressive antibiotic therapy and orbital decompression.

CT of preseptal inflammation shows a diffuse increase in density and thickening of the eyelid and conjunctiva. Abscess formation is indicated by an area of low density which may or may not exhibit rim enhancement following the administration of intravenous contrast. The globe usually does not exhibit exophthalmos and occasionally is displaced slightly posteriorly.

With subperiosteal inflammation, the exudate accumulates between the lamina papyracea and the loose periosteum. Initially this may only be a phlegmonous cellulitis, but if inadequately treated it will progress to abscess formation. The CT characteristics are similar for both subperiosteal phlegmon and subperiosteal abscess. The medial rectus muscle is displaced laterally, is broadened due to inflammatory edema and may enhance slightly. The elevated periosteum is displaced laterally and is demonstrated as an enhancing line running alongside the medial rectus muscle. The thickened periosteum may be indistinguishable from the medial rectus muscle. An abscess becomes apparent by the development of an area of low density which may be localized or spread along the entire medial wall of the orbit. The inflammation may cause demineralization of the lamina papyracea or even osteitis which becomes evident with bony loss or thinning (Figures 8.15 and 8.16).

Usually the infection is limited by the periosteum and it rarely spreads into the intraconal space. Should spread occur, the fat in the intraconal space is infiltrated with linear strands of inflammatory reaction, making it difficult to distinguish either the extraocular muscles or the optic nerve. Abscess formation is indicated by the characteristic development of an area of low density with an enhancing rim (Figures 8.16 and 8.17).

Intracranial complications

These are the rare but life-threatening complications of uncontrolled sinus disease and include meningitis, extradural abscess, intradural abscess, subdural abscess, intracerebral abscess and cavernous sinus thrombosis. Such complications usually occur as a consequence of inadequate antibiotic treatment, the presence of resistant bacteria or immunosuppression. The infection may spread by one of several routes:

i   direct spread if the infected sinus is involved in trauma;
ii   through congenital bony dehiscences, such as defects in the wall of the sphenoid sinus;
iii by retrograde phlebitis;
iv   through erosion of the bony wall by infection or tumor;
v   by hematogenous spread as part of a generalized septicemia;
vi   by extension along pre-existing anatomic pathways, i.e. perineurally along the olfactory nerves or via nerves that communicate into the pterygopalatine fossa, the vidian nerve or the maxillary division of the trigeminal nerve.

The clinical features of intracranial sepsis may at first be nonspecific and include malaise and generalized headache. As the clinical picture develops, the symptoms depend on the site of the intracranial infection. A high index of suspicion is needed to make the appropriate diagnosis and arrest the infection before serious neurologic sequelae occur. The headache becomes more severe with progression of the infection. Focal signs and convulsions may occur as well as changes in personality and conscious level. Vomiting and papilledema occur at a late stage. Examination of the cerebrospinal fluid may be of value in identifying elevated protein and leukocyte levels and reduced glucose levels, as well as providing information after bacteriological culture. However, CT is invaluable in identifying if and where an intracranial abscess has occurred.

If meningitis is localized to the base of the skull, multiple cranial nerve palsies may present. Obstruction to the flow of cerebrospinal fluid leads to dilation of the ventricles and hydrocephalus. Cortical and gyral enhancement may be seen following the administration of intravenous contrast.

An extradural abscess occurs between the bone of the calvarium and the dura mater. CT will usually demonstrate a collection that is lentiform in shape and will be limited by the dural attachment to the suture lines between the individual skull bones (Figure 6.18). The adjacent brain is usually hypodense because the surrounding tissue is edematous. If an abscess forms in the subdural space, i.e. between the dura and the arachnoid, it tends to have a semilunar shape. It may extend into the interhemispheric fissures or along the margins of the tentorium. Both the periosteum and the meninges will enhance following the administration of intravenous contrast. The collection of pus will vary in density depending on the contents and how long the abscess has been present. Air may be seen in the fluid collection.

An intracerebral abscess may result from the direct spread of infection from the sinus into the cerebral tissue, or following septic embolization. In the former situation the abscess is usually in close proximity to the infected sinus responsible, whereas in the latter situation the abscess may be distant to the infected sinus. Infection of the frontal sinus is frequently responsible for intracerebral abscesses, and these may reach some size before the diagnosis becomes clinically evident. The CT findings will vary depending on the stage of development that the abscess has reached at the time of the scan. Early in the abscess formation there may be only a poorly defined hypodense area exhibiting little enhancement. If untreated, this will progress to exhibit a well-demarcated, encapsulated lesion surrounding an area of pus. The capsule enhances brightly following intravenous contrast administration, and the surrounding brain appears hypodense reflecting the edema in the region.

Cavernous sinus thrombosis is a further rare intracranial complication of sinusitis. Acute thrombophlebitis secondary to infection in an area with venous drainage into the cavernous sinus, such as acute sphenoiditis, is the usual predisposing factor. The clinical features include fever, headache and rigors. There is edema of the eyelids, exophthalmos, chemosis, ophthalmoplegia, and low-grade papilledema. The white cell count is elevated and blood culture is often positive.

On CT a normal cavernous sinus is seen to as a brightly enhancing structure surrounding the pituitary fossa, with a sharply defined lateral border. Usually the intracavernous part of the internal carotid artery is indistinguishable from the surrounding venous structure. In contrast, in cavernous sinus thrombosis the venous structure fails to enhance and the internal carotid arteries will become very prominent as enhanced tubular structure.

NASAL POLYPS

The etiology of nasal polyps remains unclear. Chronic inflammation, be it allergic or infective, results in hyperplasia and edema of the sinonasal mucosa. There is accumulation of fluid in the stroma of the polyps due to a deranged vascular mechanism. The cellularity of the polyps varies and eosinophils are predominant in polyps derived from allergic or atopic patients.

Clinically these patients present with a long history of nasal obstruction, rhinorrhea, recurrent sinusitis and/or headaches. Rarely, hypertelorism or exophthalmos may be found on examination. Both the nasal cavities are usually filled with multiple polyps, and the finding of a unilateral polyp should raise the suspicion of tumor or even malignancy.

Endoscopically it has been shown that most of the polyps appearing in the nasal cavity arise from the ethmoidal area. The most frequent sites of origin are the areas of contact between the infundibulum, the middle turbinate and the uncinate process (Figures 8.19–8.21). In many patients, polyps arise from the anterior aspect of the ethmoid bulla and protrude into the middle meatus. In up to 50% of patients, polyps are found in the frontal recess (Figure 8.22). Polyps have also been identified arising in a concha bullosa and in the lateral recess. The latter is most frequently affected when there is simultaneous polypoid involvement of the posterior ethmoid sinus (Figures 8.23 and 8.24). In uncomplicated polyposis, the anterior ethmoid is almost always involved; isolated polyps have not been identified arising solely from the posterior ethmoid sinus, except around tumor. Only 8% of sphenoid sinuses show any polypoid change. Relatively minor polypoid change in the ostiomeatal complex revealed by diagnostic endoscopy may be found to be extensive when the patient is examined by CT.

Plain radiographs of patients with diffuse nasal polyposis show nonspecific changes. There is often widespread loss of translucence from mucosal thickening, sinus opacification and, occasionally, evidence of bony expansion in the ethmoid sinuses.

The findings on CTs are of unilateral or bilateral soft-tissue masses within the nasal cavity and paranasal sinuses. These are usually of alternating mucoid density and soft-tissue density, which becomes more marked on examination with narrow-window settings (Figures 8.25 and 8.26). If the polyps are tightly packed together there may be resorption of the ethmoid bony leaflets (Figure 8.27). This is represented by areas of high density surrounded by areas of mucoid density. In other cases, the bony leaflets may become sclerotic and make a more definite impression on the image (Figures 8.28 and 8.29). Sometimes, following intravenous administration, slightly enhancing curvilinear looping strands will be seen in the diseased area. This represents areas of mucous membrane surrounded by the mucoid material within the polyp. This becomes more apparent if the scans are examined with narrow-window settings. If the polyps are longstanding, there may be hypertelorism and smooth expansion of the bony walls of the sinuses secondary to pressure effects.

It may be difficult to accurately interpret CTs of patients with massive polyposis if they have undergone previous surgery. There may be extensive resorption of bone following pressure necrosis and all that may be seen is an amorphous mass of disease indicating the need for radical procedure, which may be at variance to the decision based on the diagnostic endoscopy (Figures 8.30 and 8.31). Surgical decisions should not be based solely on the radiographic findings. However, in those who have undergone previous surgery, CT is of value in determining the presence of any bony defects at critical points and the site of recurrent polyps which may be attached to the dura.

There are no unique radiologic features that will lead to a definite diagnosis of polyposis. In view of the bone resorption that may occur, a tissue biopsy must always be taken to exclude malignancy. The associated bony sclerosis may be suggestive of a chronic inflammatory process, but it is also associated with inverting papilloma. The internal architecture of the polypoid mass helps to differentiate it from a mucocele which is usually non-enhancing and isodense, being filled with fluid of uniform density (Figures 8.32 and 8.33). The finding of mixed density or the alternating radiating bands of high and low density associated with polyposis may lead to suspicion of a fungal sinusitis. However, bilateral and extensive involvement is an unusual feature of fungal sinusitis (Figures 8.26–8.28) in an otherwise healthy patient, unless the patient has allergic fungal sinusitis.

ANTROCHOANAL POLYPS

The etiology of these unilateral polyps is unclear, although they are histologically similar to ordinary inflammatory nasal polyps. An antrochoanal sinus, which originates most commonly from the posterolateral wall, and a solid part that extends by a stalk through the maxillary ostium or via an accessory ostium in the anterior or posterior nasal fontanelles, into the middle meatus, which progressively expands to reach the choana. Antrochoanal polyps occur more frequently in children and young adults and have a tendency to recur if inadequately excised.

The radiographic appearance on plain radiographs shows a homogenous area in the maxillary sinus which reflects the cystic component, and an opaque nasal cavity. A lateral view may demonstrate the smooth posterior margin of the polyps hanging in the nasopharynx. The CT demonstrates on opaque maxillary sinus of uniform density, with a soft-tissue mass in the ipsilateral nasal cavity. The sinus ostium and the nasal cavity may be widened to accommodate the polyp (Figure 8.34). Occasionally the surrounding bone may exhibit a mixture of resorption and reactive osteitis. The differential diagnosis includes hemangioma, juvenile angiofibroma and inverting papilloma, as well as any other relatively slow-growing malignancy.

RETENTION CYSTS

These benign cysts have multiple causes, including trauma infection and allergy (Figure 8.35). They occur following obstruction of either a minor salivary gland or a mucus-secreting gland. The former, nonsecretory cysts consist of serous fluid which forms loculated collections in the connective tissue of the mucous membrane. The cyst has no definable lining. The mucus-secreting cyst is lined with respiratory epithelium: it is usually asymptomatic and presents as an incidental finding on 2–5% of radiographs of the facial region. The radiographic features are of a dome-shaped density, usually arising in the floor of the sinus (Figure 8.36). However cysts may arise at any mucosal site (Figures 8.37–8.39). The surrounding anatomy is usually normal unless the cyst is of a large dimension, when some bone remodeling may occur. If the cyst fills the sinus cavity, a crescentic rim of air above the cyst usually allows one to differentiate the cyst from a mucocele. Retention cysts may sit on the infraorbital nerve where it passes through the roof of the maxillary sinus, and so cause paresthesia of the infraorbital nerve. These cysts rarely need any treatment, but when they are observed it is important to make certain that there is no altered anatomy or paresthesia (Figure 8.37). Should this be the case,

a biopsy may be necessary to exclude sinister disease. Dental disease in the form of odontogenic cysts should also be excluded.

MUCOCELES

A mucocele is a sac containing mucus and desquamated epithelium; it completely fills the sinus and is capable of slow expansion, which may lead to compression of the adjacent structures. The causes are multifactorial and include obstruction of the ostium with chronic inflammation or polyps, trauma (surgical or accidental), allergy and tumor.

Mucoceles may occur in any sinus cavity including that of a concha bullosa. They present more commonly in the frontoethmoid complex; occasionally, multiple mucoceles may occur in the same patient (Figure 8.40). Mucoceles of the frontal sinus present with swelling of the upper eyelid and inferior displacement of the globe. There may also be swelling over the anterior wall of the frontal sinus with the characteristic 'eggshell crackling' on palpation. Mucoceles of the ethmoid sinus tend to cause exophthalmos and lateral displacement of the globe. There may be an associated swelling in the superomedial quadrant of the orbit and both these features may cause diplopia. Encroachment on the lacrimal apparatus causes epiphora. Sphenoid sinus mucoceles tend to present with headache or retroorbital or periorbital pain. They may expand into the cavernous sinus and the orbital apex causing ophthalmoplegia and retroorbital pain known as the 'orbital apex syndrome'. There may be an associated gradual loss of vision, papilledema and optic atrophy. These patients can also present with multiple cranial nerve palsies. Mucoceles of the maxillary sinus may present in many ways; as a mass in the nasal cavity if there is medial extension, with diplopia if there is superior extension, with cheek swelling if there is anterior expansion and swelling of the gums if there is extension into the alveolus (Figures 8.41–8.43). A significant number of maxillary sinus mucoceles follow surgical procedures on the maxillary sinus, and these are characteristically found to be laterally placed in the sinus as opposed to filling the entire antrum (Figure 8.44). Rarely, mucoceles of the lacrimal sac may occur. These usually occur in infants and present with a swelling in the region of the medial canthus. These are usually related to congenital anomalies of the nasolacrimal duct.

Clinical examination and plain radiographs may indicate the diagnosis. For confirmation of the diagnosis and delineation of the extent of the mucocele, CT is invaluable. The early radiologic features of a mucocele are nonspecific in comparison with those of allergy or inflammatory disease. However, as the mucus accumulates within the sinus, there is gradual expansion of the sinus cavity, with thinning and loss of the peripheral bony margins. Later, this bone remodeling will change to bony destruction and malignancy will enter the differential diagnosis. The contents of the mucocele usually appear homogenous and are isodense or hypodense relative to brain tissue. They do not usually enhance following administration of intravenous contrast. Should the mucocele become acutely infected, and develop into a pyocele, the administration of intravenous contrast will demonstrate rim enhancement. While poorly demonstrating bony defects, MR imaging has superior ability in differentiating contrast between soft tissue and it may help in the differentiation of mucoceles and solid tumors. On MR imaging, the signal intensity of mucoceles varies according to the number of hydrogen protons and glycoprotein complexes present with the mucocele.

Frontal sinus mucoceles cause erosion of the incomplete septa normally found within the sinus cavity. This leads to loss of the normal scalloped appearance and gives rise to a smooth outline. There may be an associated reactive sclerosis of the bone. With increased expansion, the anterior and posterior bony walls of the sinus may become dehiscent, risking intracranial extension and sepsis or escape of the mucocele into the upper eyelid (Figures 8.45–8.51).

Ethmoid mucoceles are difficult to diagnose on plain radiographs. they may be either radiolucent or slightly opaque. Supraorbital extension may be indicated by thinning or loss of the superomedial orbital rim and the adjacent roof of the orbit. CT will demonstrate expansion of the ethmoid sinus and loss of the fine bony septa dividing the air cells (Figures 8.40 and 8.52). The lamina papyracea may be displaced laterally and may be deficient in parts (Figures 8.53–8.55).

The polypoid mucocele is a separate entity which has been described in the ethmoid sinus. Patients with this pathology present with diplopia and exophthalmos. It exhibits involvement and expansion of the whole ethmoid labyrinth with preservation and sclerosis of the lamina papyracea and the bony leaflets separating the ethmoid air cells (Figures 8.54 and 8.55). These lesions have also been noted to enhance slightly following the administration of intravenous contrast, which is at variance to the behavior of the classic mucocele. These polypoid mucoceles are usually associated with multiple sinus inflammatory disease and not infrequently with other mucoceles developing in the supraorbital ethmoid air cells.

Sphenoid sinus mucoceles may be localized unilaterally within the sinus or may expand to fill the whole sinus. Early features include a hemispherical opacity of the sinus. There may be displacement of the intersinus septum and the lesion may then spread into the posterior ethmoid and the sphenoethmoid recess. If extensive the mucocele will be seen expanding into any of the related anatomic regions, for example, into the cranial cavity, nasopharynx, pterygopalatine fossa, infratemporal fossa or orbit. The latter may be associated with widening of the superior orbital fissure. This extensive appearance may be suggestive of malignancy.

Maxillary sinus mucoceles in the early stage will exhibit opacification of the sinus on plain radiographs. As the mucocele expands, the bony walls become thinned and displaced medially into the nasal cavity, superiorly into the orbit, posteriorly into the pterygopalatine fossa or laterally reversing the natural convexity of the lateral antral wall (Figures 8.41, 8.42 and 8.56). If the patient has had surgery to the maxillary sinus, the mucocele may be lateralized within a small compartment and the surrounding wall may be sclerotic (Figure 8.44). The density of the fluid is less than that of muscle and isodense with brain. The differential diagnosis includes malignancy, especially if bony erosion is present.

Lacrimal sac mucoceles are an uncommon finding in infants. CT is an invaluable aid to confirming the diagnosis as it will demonstrate a cystic mass in the medial canthus in continuity with an expanded nasolacrimal duct and a contiguous submucosal intranasal mass.

PYOCELE

A pyocele is a mucocele that has become secondarily infected. This usually exacerbates the symptoms. The radiologic features are similar to those of mucoceles, but following the administration of intravenous contrast there is usually a ring of enhancement within the cavity of the pyocele, representing the inflamed mucosa (Figure 8.57).

ATROPHIC RHINITIS

Atrophic rhinitis is a poorly understood condition which is characterized by atrophy of the nasal mucosa and reabsorption of the underlying bone. The lateral nasal wall becomes bowed and therefore the nasal cavity becomes enlarged. This process is usually symmetrical, but may occur unilaterally. Despite the greater dimensions of the nasal cavity, these patients usually complain of nasal obstruction. Other clinical features include anosmia and an offensive purulent rhinorrhea. Atrophic rhinitis may occur as a primary disease of the nasal cavity or it may follow intranasal surgery.

On CTs, there are characteristic findings associated with atrophic rhinitis. These include bony resorption and mucosal atrophy of the inferior and middle turbinates, enlargement of the nasal cavity with lateral bowing of the lateral nasal wall, hypoplasia of the maxillary sinuses, bony resorption of the ethmoid bulla and ethmoid sinuses, loss of definition of the ostiomeatal complex, and mucosal thickening in the paranasal sinuses (Figures 8.58 and 8.59).

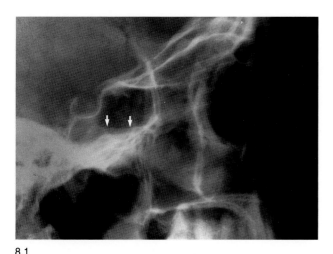

8.1

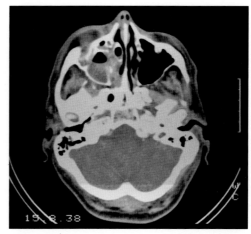

8.2

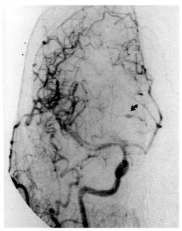
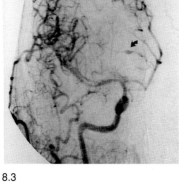

8.3

8.4

Figure **8.1**

Acute sphenoid sinusitis. An upright lateral plain radiograph of the paranasal sinuses demonstrates an air–fluid level in the sphenoid sinus consistent with acute sphenoid sinusitis (arrows).

Figure **8.2**

Mucormycosis. This axial CT scan demonstrates sinusitis involving the right maxillary and ethmoid sinuses in addition to cellulitis of the right orbit. This patient was an uncontrolled diabetic who had undergone root canal therapy 4 days previously.

Figure **8.3**

Mucormycosis. This angiogram was obtained after an intracranial hemorrhage was identified on the CT scan of the patient shown in Figure 8.2. Note the mycotic aneurysm (arrow) which is the most likely cause of the intracranial hemorrhage.

Figure **8.4**

Chronic maxillary sinusitis: CT scan. A large retention cyst or polyp can be seen in the left maxillary sinus. There is mucosal thickening in the right maxillary sinus.

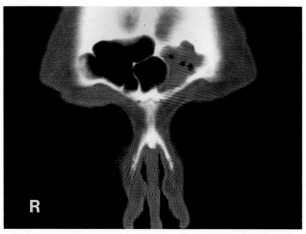

8.5

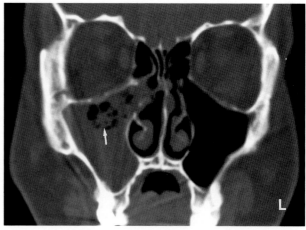

8.6

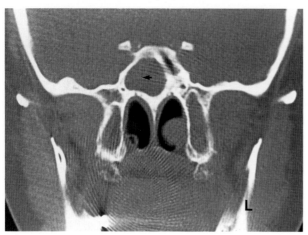

8.7

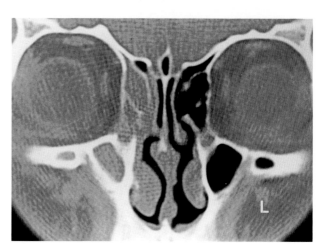

8.8

Figure **8.5**

Frontal sinusitis. This coronal CT scan demonstrates some mucous in the left frontal sinus containing characteristic bubbles of air. The right frontal sinus is well developed.

Figure **8.6**

Maxillary sinusitis. This coronal CT scan demonstrates mucosal disease with fluid in the maxillary sinus and an area of characteristic of mucous discharge in the maxillary sinus (arrow).

Figure **8.7**

Sphenoid sinusitis. This coronal CT scan demonstrates chronic sphenoid sinusitis with reactive osteitis of the sinus walls (arrow). Sphenoid sinusitis occurs more frequently than it is appreciated. These patients are more often investigated for the cause of headache by neurologists with routine head scans.

Figure **8.8**

Pansinusitis. This coronal CT scan demonstrates unilateral maxillary sinusitis and inflammatory disease in the frontal recess.

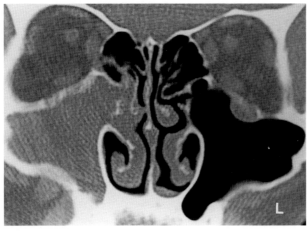

8.9

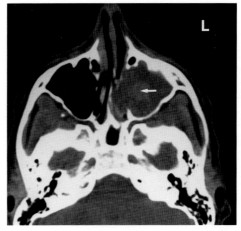

8.10

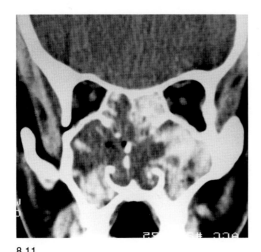

8.11

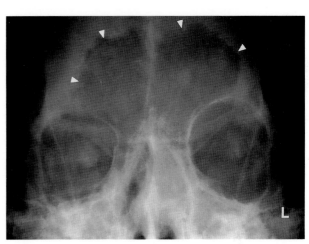

8.12

Figure **8.9**

Pansinusitis. This coronal CT scan, taken more posteriorly than Figure 8.6, demonstrates right maxillary sinusitis which also involves the anterior ethmoid sinus. There is some sclerosis of the lateral maxillary sinus wall and the floor of the orbit.

Figure **8.10**

Fungal (*Aspergillus*) sinusitis. This axial CT scan demonstrates fluid filling the entire left maxillary sinus lumen and a mass is seen causing smooth expansion of the medial sinus wall. The high-density mass noted in the lumen (arrow) of the maxillary sinus was subsequently proven to be aspergillosis.

Figure **8.11**

Fungal (*Aspergillus*) sinusitis. This CT scan demonstrates inflammatory reaction in the sinuses. The high-density areas are the result of heavy metal accumulation in the mycelia.

Figure **8.12**

Osteomyelitis. This plain radiograph demonstrates extensive destruction of the frontal bone (arrowheads) with opacification of the frontal and the ethmoid sinuses, consistent with frontoethmoid sinusitis and osteomyelitis.

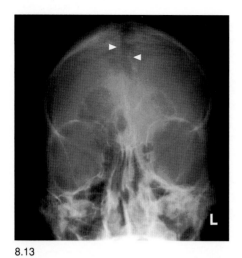

8.13

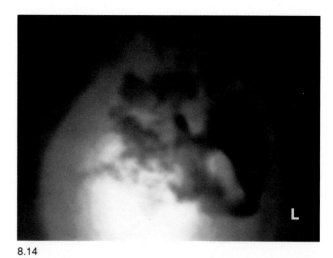

8.14

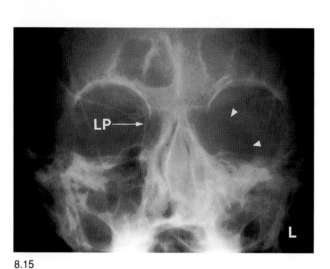

8.15

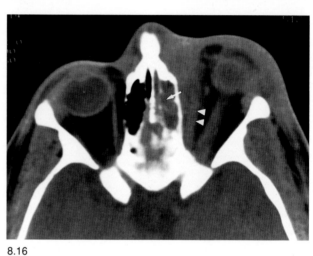

8.16

Figure **8.13**

Osteomyelitis. This plain radiograph demonstrates left-sided frontal sinusitis, with rarefaction progressing along the sagittal suture (arrowheads).

Figure **8.14**

Osteomyelitis: CT scan. This patient presented with acute frontal sinusitis which progressed to osteomyelitis. Widespread lytic lesions are seen in the frontal bone.

Figure **8.15**

Orbital cellulitis on radiograph. This patient presented with facial and orbital cellulitis, fever and a high white cell count. This Water's view demonstrates extensive destruction of the medial wall of the left orbit, destruction of the floor of the orbit and a subperiosteal abscess extending into the left orbit (arrowheads). The left maxillary, frontal and ethmoid sinuses are opaque. An air fluid level is seen in the right frontal sinus consistent with an acute right frontal sinusitis. The intact lamina papyracea is marked (LP) on the right. The patient refused to cooperate for CT.

Figure **8.16**

Subperiosteal abscess: CT. The non-enhancing mass along the medial aspect of the left ethmoid complex (arrow) is a subperiosteal abscess. The medial rectus muscle and the elevated periosteum (arrowheads) are seen as an enhancing linear density lateral to the abscess. This abscess is the result of the spread of infection from the ethmoid sinus through the lamina papyracea.

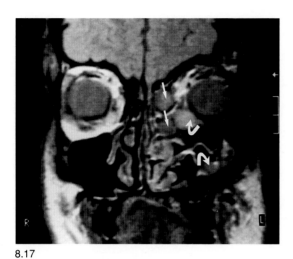

8.17

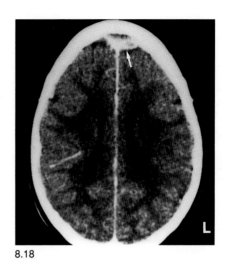

8.18

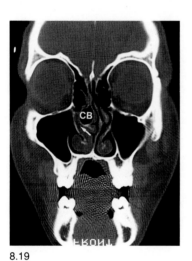

8.19

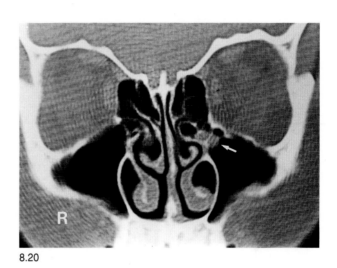

8.20

Figure **8.17**

Mucopyocele and orbital cellulitis. On this T2-weighted MR scan the signal-void masses are the mucoceles (arrows). The hypointense masses are the infected pyoceles (curved arrows); normal signal intensity is seen on the other side. Orbital fat is altered due to orbital cellulitis on the left side.

Figure **8.18**

Epidural abscess: CT. This patient presented with acute frontal sinusitis which rapidly progressed to osteomyelitis. A small epidural abscess (arrow) developed adjacent to the infected sinus, as can be seen on this CT.

Figure **8.19**

Solitary polyp. This coronal CT scan demonstrates a large polyp wedged in the middle meatus (arrow). The large concha bullosa (CB) which compromises the middle meatus is the most likely cause of the polypoid degeneration of the mucosa in the middle meatus.

Figure **8.20**

Solitary polyp. This coronal CT scan demonstrates a small polyp in the left ethmoid infundibulum (arrow). Although easily demonstrated on the scan, the polyp could not be identified on clinical examination.

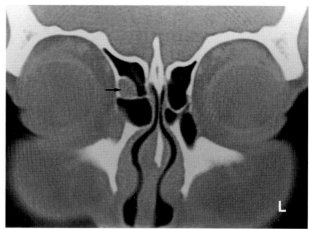

8.21

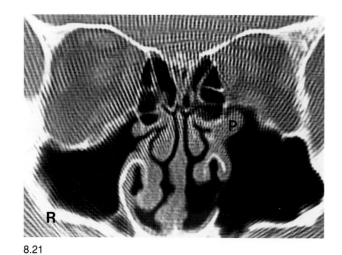

8.22

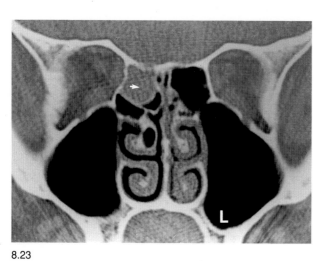

8.23

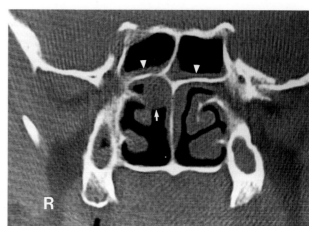

8.24

Figure **8.21**

Solitary polyp. This coronal CT scan demonstrates occlusion of the left maxillary ostium by a solitary polyp (P). Despite a previous intranasal antrostomy the patient had remained symptomatic.

Figure **8.22**

Solitary polyp. This coronal CT scan demonstrates a soft-tissue density above the right agger nasi cell in the frontal recess (arrow). The adjacent lamina papyracea is intact and normal. This transpired to be an inflammatory polyp.

Figure **8.23**

Nasal polyps. This coronal CT scan demonstrates a solitary polyp (arrow) in the right posterior ethmoid air cell or Onodi's cell.

Figure **8.24**

Nasal polyps. This posterior coronal CT scan demonstrates inflammatory mucosal thickening in the sphenoid sinuses (arrowheads), as well as a polyp arising in the right sphenoethmoid recess (arrow).

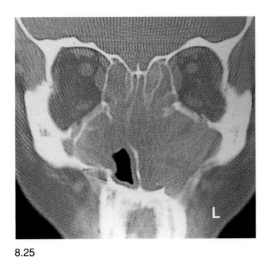

8.25

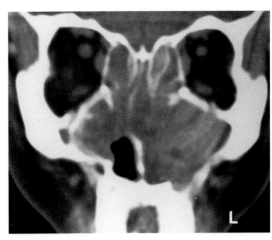

8.26

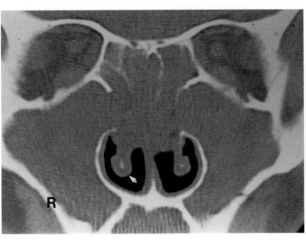

8.27

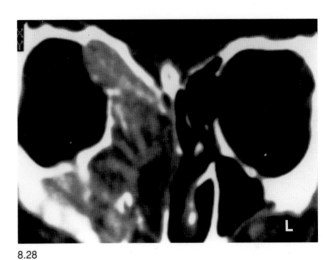

8.28

Figure **8.25**

Nasal polyposis. This coronal CT scan, examined with a wide window, demonstrates that the maxillary sinuses, the anterior ethmoid sinuses and the nasal cavity are occluded by either soft-tissue or fluid-filled densities.

Figure **8.26**

Nasal polyposis. This coronal CT scan, examined with a narrow window, demonstrates that the soft-tissue abnormality has the alternating high- and low-density areas characteristic of benign nasal polyposis. The alternating features are due to the mixture of high-density mucoid material and low-density fluid.

Figure **8.27**

Nasal polyposis. This coronal CT scan demonstrates extensive polyposis occluding the entire nasal cavity. The plane of demarcation between the lateral nasal wall and the maxillary sinus is indistinct. The inferior turbinates are small and shrunken from chronic abuse of topical decongestants (arrow).

Figure **8.28**

Nasal polyposis. This coronal CT scan, examined with a narrow window, demonstrates benign nasal polyps associated with a mucocele in the ethmoid sinus following obstruction of the ostia. The alternating densities are due to the mucoid material in the polyp (low density) and the dense mucosal folds. The superomedial margin of the orbit is eroded.

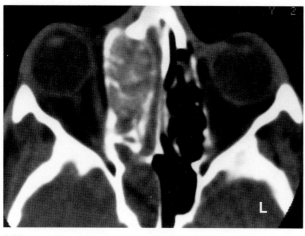

8.29

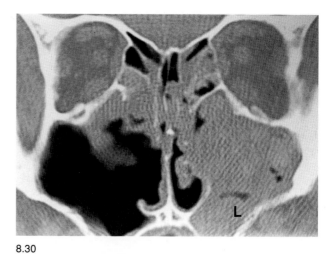

8.30

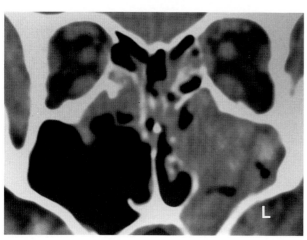

8.31

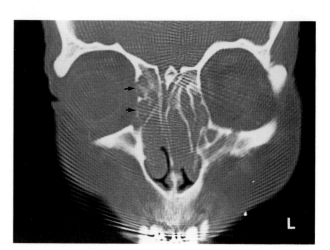

8.32

Figure **8.29**

Nasal polyposis. This narrow-window axial CT scan of the same patient as in Figure 8.28, demonstrates widening of the ethmoid labyrinth into the right orbit with preservation of the bony septa that separate the ethmoid air cells. This has some of the features of an ethmoid polypoid mucocele. The lamina papyracea is thickened and sclerotic.

Figure **8.30**

Recurrent nasal polyps. This coronal CT scan, examined with a wide window demonstrates the defect of a radical drainage procedure conducted for chronic maxillary sinusitis. The medial wall of the maxillary sinus, the middle and inferior turbinates on the right side have been removed. The remainder of the sinuses are filled with apparently homogenous soft tissue.

Figure **8.31**

Recurrent nasal polyps. This narrow-window coronal CT scan of the same patient as in Figure 8.30 demonstrates alternating high and low densities in the left maxillary sinus, consistent with recurrent polypoid tissue.

Figure **8.32**

Polypoidal mucocele. This coronal CT scan demonstrates extensive soft tissue filling the ethmoid air cells. The bony erosion seen in the right lamina papyracea (arrows) raises the possibility of either polypoid disease or a mucocele. The smooth expansion characteristic of a mucocele is absent.

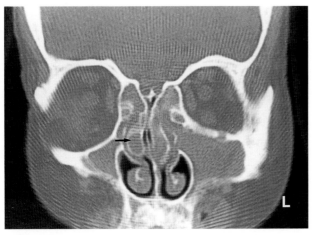

8.33

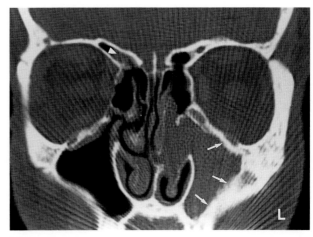

8.34

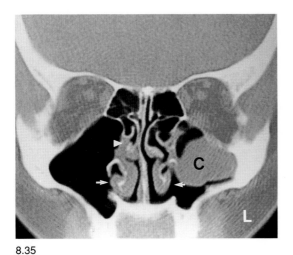

8.35

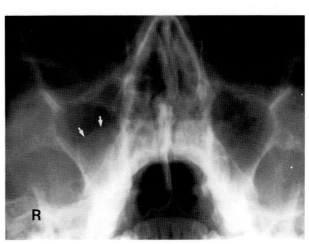

8.36

Figure **8.33**

Polypoidal mucocele. This coronal CT scan is more posterior than that in Figure 8.32. The extensive soft tissue seen throughout the paranasal sinuses was due to polypoidal disease. There is a diseased concha bullosa on the right (arrow).

Figure **8.34**

Antrochoanal polyp. This coronal CT scan demonstrates a large inflammatory antrochoanal polyp that extends from the left maxillary sinus into the middle meatus. Chronic inflammation has resulted in extensive reactive osteitis and thickening of the left lateral maxillary sinus wall and orbital floor (arrows). A small polyp is demonstrated in the right frontal recess (arrowhead).

Figure **8.35**

Mucous retention cyst. This coronal CT scan demonstrates bilateral intranasal antrostomies (arrows) despite which the patient continues to be symptomatic. There remains bilateral ostiomeatal complex disease with inflammatory disease in the right middle meatus (arrowhead). A small retention cyst or polyp is seen within the lumen of the left maxillary sinus (C). Most cysts are situated in the dependent part of the sinus cavity.

Figure **8.36**

Mucous retention cyst. Radiograph: this Water's view demonstrates a dome-shaped soft-tissue filling defect arising from the floor of the right maxillary sinus (arrows).

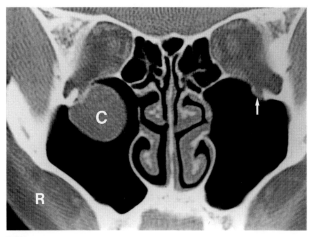

8.37

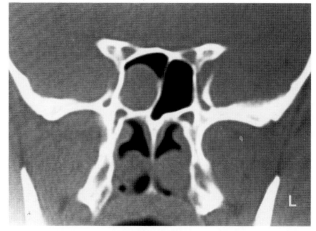

8.38

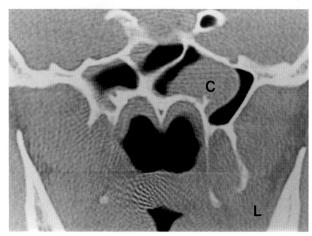

8.39

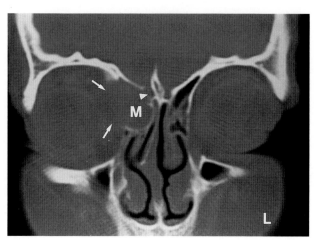

8.40

Figure **8.37**

Mucous retention cyst. This coronal CT scan demonstrates a mucous retention cyst (C) adjacent to the right infraorbital canal. The left infraorbital canal is demonstrated (arrow).

Figure **8.38**

Mucous retention cyst. This coronal CT scan demonstrates a large cyst or polyp arising in the right sphenoid sinus.

Figure **8.39**

Mucous retention cyst. This coronal CT scan demonstrates a multiseptate sphenoid sinus with a retention cyst (C), in the left lateral recess. Note the pneumatization of the left anterior clinoid process.

Figure **8.40**

Ethmoid mucocele. This coronal CT scan demonstrates an isodense soft-tissue mass with expansion and erosion of the ethmoid fovea (arrowhead) and the superomedial margin of the orbit (arrows). This has the features of a mucocele (M). The scan also demonstrates the limited surgical access as a result of encroachment of the middle turbinate and of the deviated nasal septum onto the middle meatus. The arrowhead demonstrates the erosion of the ethmoid fovea.

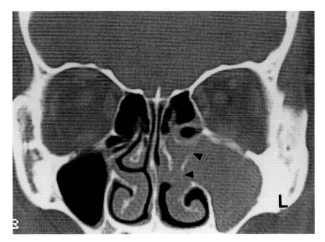

8.41

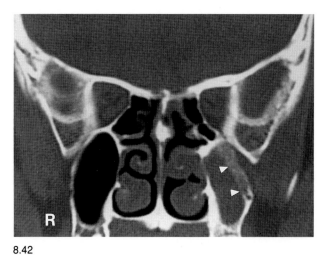

8.42

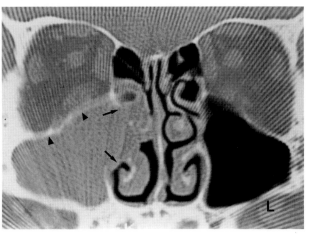

8.43

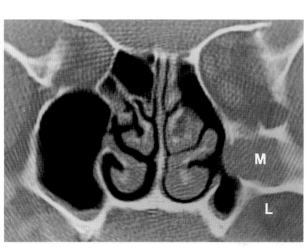

8.44

Figure **8.41**

Maxillary sinus mucocele. This coronal CT scan demonstrates an expansile soft-tissue density within the maxillary sinus, with bowing of the medial wall of the maxillary sinus (arrowheads).

Figure **8.43**

Maxillary sinus mucocele. This narrow-window coronal CT scan shows that the maxillary sinus cavity is filled with fluid. The secondary changes caused by mucoceles such as medial expansion of the maxillary sinus lumen (arrows), and reactive sclerosis of the orbital floor (arrowheads), are at an early stage.

Figure **8.42**

Maxillary sinus mucocele. This more posterior CT scan demonstrates irregular bony resorption in the lateral wall (arrowheads), of the maxillary sinus. This was found to be a pyocele.

Figure **8.44**

Maxillary sinus mucocele. This coronal CT scan demonstrates the bony defect from previous intranasal antrostomy. As a result of scarring, a mucocele (M), limited to the lateral compartment of the septated maxillary sinus has developed.

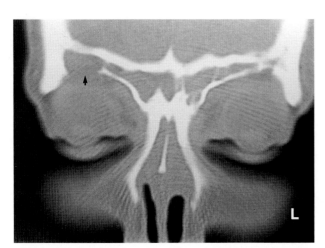

8.45

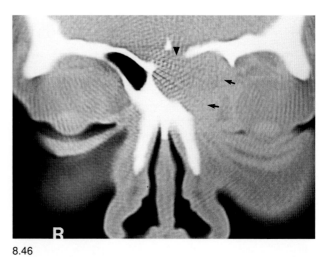

8.46

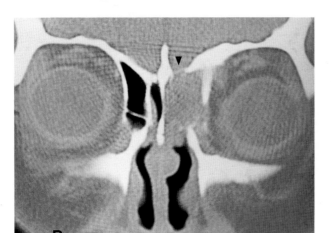

8.47

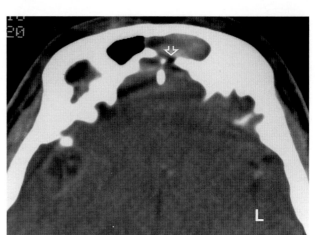

8.48

Figure **8.45**

Frontal sinus mucocele. This coronal CT scan demonstrates a defect in the floor of the right frontal sinus (arrow). The patient had polypoid disease with a small mucocele in the lateral part of the frontal sinus. This is unusual, as most frontal sinus mucoceles occur close to the superomedial margin of the orbit.

Figure **8.46**

Left frontoethmoid mucocele. This patient had previously undergone sinus surgery for chronic sinusitis and presented with a mass in the superomedial aspect of the orbit. This coronal CT scan demonstrates a smooth, expansile, soft-tissue mass with erosion of both cribriform plates (arrowheads), and the superomedial aspect of the orbit (arrows). This mucocele developed after scarring occluded drainage of the frontal recess on the left side.

Figure **8.47**

Left frontoethmoid mucocele. This coronal CT scan was taken posterior to Figure 8.46 and demonstrates a smooth, expansile, soft-tissue mass, with erosion of the left lamina papyracea and the left cribriform plate (arrowhead). The soft-tissue images of the orbital contents show the globe to be displaced inferolaterally on the left.

Figure **8.48**

Frontoethmoid pyomucocele. This axial CT scan demonstrates an expansile, soft-tissue mass which has eroded through the posterior wall of the frontal sinus (open arrow). There is enhancement of the mucous membrane consistent with a pyomucocele of the left frontal sinus.

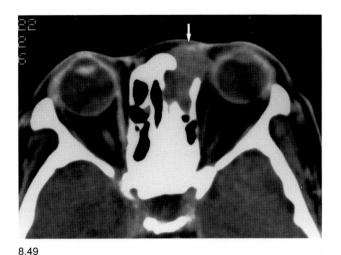

8.49

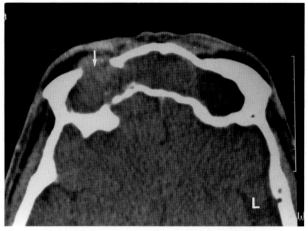

8.50

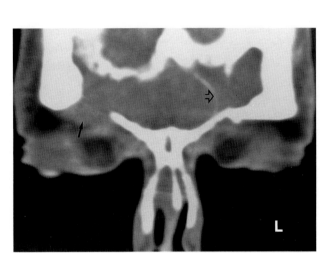

8.51

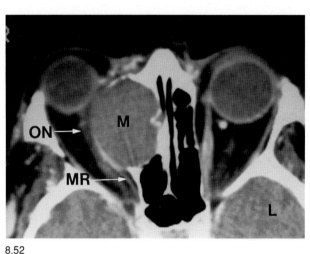

8.52

Figure **8.49**

Frontoethmoid pyomucocele. This axial CT scan demonstrates an expansile, soft-tissue mass which has eroded through the anterior margin of the ethmoid sinus (arrow). There is enhancement of the mucous membrane in keeping with a pyomucocele of the ethmoid sinuses.

Figure **8.50**

Frontal mucocele. This axial CT scan demonstrates an enhancing mass which has eroded the anterior wall of the frontal sinus (arrow). Reactive sclerosis of the sinus walls is noted. This was a frontal sinus mucocele. If erosion is the dominant feature, a mucocele may be difficult to differentiate radiologically from a malignant tumor.

Figure **8.51**

Frontal sinus mucocele. This coronal CT scan, of the same patient in Figure 8.50 demonstrates the laterally placed frontal sinus mucocele, with erosion of the floor of the lateral part of the sinus (arrow). The intersinus septum is bowed to the left (open arrow).

Figure **8.52**

Ethmoid mucocele. CT scan: this patient presented with right-sided exophthalmos. A smooth expansile mass (M) with thinning of the lamina papyracea is seen in the right ethmoid sinus. The medial rectus (MR) muscle is stretched over the mucocele. The smooth margins and erosions suggest the presence of a mucocele. The optic nerve (ON) is displaced laterally.

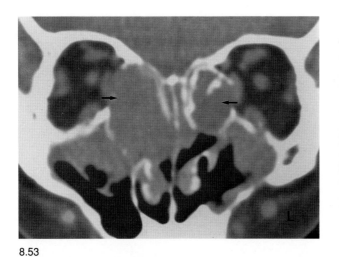

8.53

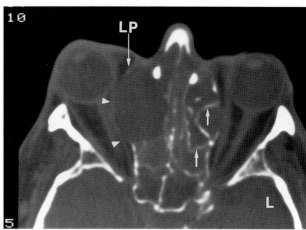

8.54

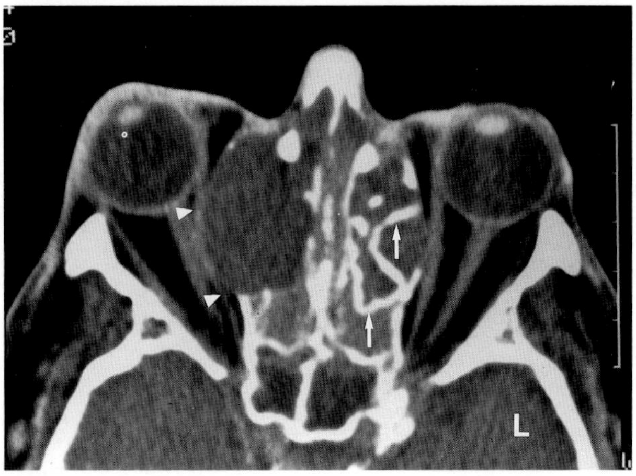

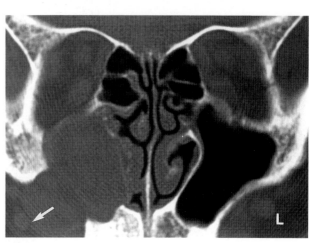

8.55

8.56

Figure **8.53**

Multiple mucoceles. This patient has undergone multiple sinus operations. The coronal CT scan demonstrates large bilateral ethmoid sinus mucoceles (arrows) with expansion and erosion of the wall of the ethmoid and frontal sinuses and the lamina papyracea.

Figure **8.54**

Ethmoid sinus polypoidal mucoceles with bilateral exophthalmos. This axial CT scan demonstrates a smooth expansile mass in the right ethmoid sinus, with eggshell thinning of the lamina papyracea (LP). The bony septa in the left ethmoid sinus are sclerotic (arrows) and the labyrinth is expanded in keeping with the diagnosis of a polypoid mucocele. The right medial rectus muscle is stretched over the mucocele (arrowheads).

Figure **8.55**

Ethmoid sinus polypoidal mucoceles with bilateral exophthalmos. This narrow-window axial CT scan of the same patient as Figure 8.54 demonstrates the smooth, expansile mass in the right ethmoid sinus to be isodense. The bony septa in the left ethmoid sinus appear sclerotic (arrows) and the labyrinth is expanded in keeping with the diagnosis of a polypoid mucocele. The right medial rectus muscle is stretched over the mucocele (arrowheads).

Figure **8.56**

Maxillary sinus mucocele. This patient presented with a mass in the right cheek (arrow). The wide-window coronal CT scan demonstrates a large, expansile mass in the right maxillary sinus which is of similar density to water. Smooth expansion of the maxillary sinus with erosion of the inferolateral wall and the roof of the maxillary sinus has occurred.

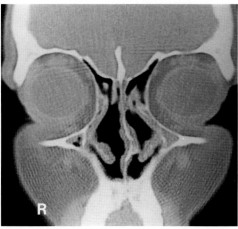

8.57

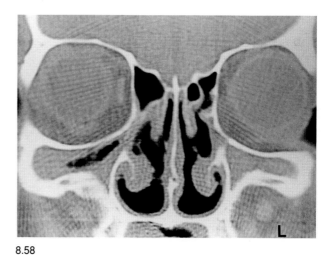

8.58

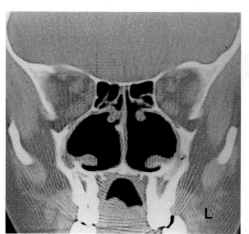

8.59A

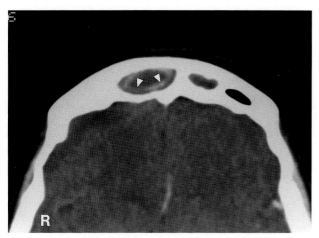

8.59B

Figure **8.57**

Pyocele. This patient presented with a furuncle on the forehead which developed into a draining sinus. Following the administration of intravenous contrast, CT demonstrates mucosal enhancement (arrowheads) in the frontal sinus. The mucosal enhancement is suggestive of an acute inflammatory process. The erosion through the anterior wall of the frontal sinus, not demonstrated on this scan, was the drainage pathway of the pyocele.

Figure **8.58**

Atrophic rhinitis. This coronal CT scan demonstrates inflammatory mucosal thickening in both maxillary sinuses. The middle and inferior turbinates have atrophied and there are few bony septa in the ethmoid labyrinth. The nasal cavities appear to be enlarged.

Figure **8.59**

Atrophic rhinitis. These coronal CT scans demonstrate expanded nasal cavities due to the resorption of both the turbinates and the bony walls of the nasal cavities. There has been a proportionate decrease in the volume of the adjacent paranasal sinuses. Despite the spacious nasal cavities, these patients often complain of nasal obstruction.

9

The radiologic appearance of tumors and tumor-like conditions of the paranasal sinuses

BENIGN TUMORS

Osteoma

Osteomas are benign, slowly growing tumors containing mature compact or cancellous bone. They occur most frequently in the frontal sinus (Figure 9.1), followed by the ethmoid (Figure 9.2) and then the maxillary sinuses. Osteomas are usually asymptomatic and are an incidental finding on radiographs conducted for an unrelated reason. However, should the osteoma block the drainage pathway of the sinus, then recurrent sinus infections or a mucocele may develop, and surgical excision of the osteoma is then indicated. Large frontal sinus osteomas can erode the inner table of the frontal bone and produce pneumocephalus or allow a sinus infection to spread intracranially. Rarely, if an osteoma arises in the ethmoid sinus and becomes extensive, it may present with exophthalmos, following invasion of the orbit, or visual deterioration, if the lesion extends back into the sphenoid and compromises the optic nerve. Osteomas in the maxillary sinus are an infrequent finding and are usually resected through an antrostomy.

The radiologic features are those of a diffusely dense mass that does not enhance following the administration of intravenous contrast. The bony margins are sharply defined and the mass may appear pedunculated or broadly based. Small osteomas may not be detected on routine radiographs and are best seen on computed tomography (CT) scans. As bone and air are seen as signal void areas on magnetic resonance imaging (MR), osteomas will be missed on MR.

The development of multiple osteomas may precede the development of multiple colonic polyposis in an autosomal dominant syndrome–Gardner's syndrome. Gardner's syndrome is also associated with multiple sebaceous cysts.

Fibrous dysplasia and ossifying fibroma

Fibrous dysplasia and ossifying fibroma are difficult to distinguish histologically. Both belong to a range of fibro-osseous lesions affecting the mandible, the maxilla and, occasionally, the other bones of the skull. The ossifying fibroma is usually a well-circumscribed lesion which lends itself to easy excision. The radiologic appearance is that of expansion of the affected bone with a sclerotic bony margin. There are often areas of fibrous tissue that are more extensive than those seen in fibrous dysplasia. The lesion may exhibit oval areas of fibrous or osseous tissue. With increasing maturity, these lesions exhibit increasing radiodense opacities (Figure 9.3).

Fibrous dysplasia is a development disease of bone, usually seen in childhood and adolescence; in most cases, it arises before the age of 20 years. The maxilla is affected more frequently than the mandible, and such cases usually present with bony swelling. Fibrous dysplasia may also affect the zygoma, the frontal bone (Figures 9.4–9.6), the ethmoid labyrinth and the sphenoid (Figure 9.6), causing facial deformity. Fibrous dysplasia can be monostotic or polyostotic. It may be confined to only one bone of the cranium (monostotic), in which case there will be a better chance of therapeutic success, if needed. In those cases in which multiple bones of the cranium are involved (polyostotic), the prognosis is worse. Extensive fibrous dysplasia can narrow the cranial nerve foramina, producing a sometimes severe compressive effect upon the cranial nerves.

Little treatment is required. The bone may be recontoured when there is cosmetic defect or function is compromised. Malignant change has been documented in these lesions, but it usually follows radiotherapy, which is now regarded as being of little value.

The radiologic features are characteristic of this disease process. The appearance varies depending on the quantity of fibrous tissue that is present in the newly formed osteoid. The bone appears thickened and has areas of increased density, which reflects the calcified cartilage and osteoid. The bone exhibits a 'ground-glass' texture (Figures 9.5 and 9.6) that is well demonstrated by CT. The sinus is usually expanded and the process may involve the neighboring structures, such as the orbit, cranial cavity and adjacent soft-tissue spaces.

Both ossifying fibromas and fibrous dysplasia are more clearly demonstrated using wide windows.

Dentigerous cysts

A solitary dentigerous cyst is found surrounding the crown of an unerupted permanent tooth. These are more commonly found in the mandible but they may also occur in the maxilla. Dentigerous cysts present as a rapidly growing mass, usually in a young adult, and may lead to facial asymmetry. The diagnosis is usually readily reached with the aid of plain radiographs or an orthopantomograph. If the diagnosis is in doubt, CT will delineate the anatomy clearly. There is usually a radiolucent area in the upper or lower jaw, associated with the crown of an unerupted tooth (Figure 9.7). The lesion is usually unilocular and surrounded by sclerotic bone. As the cyst grows it may drag the unerupted tooth with it (Figures 9.8 and 9.9). When the cyst erupts into the maxillary sinus it may grow rapidly while still retaining a thin lamella of bone (Figure 9.10).

Hemangioma

These intensely enhancing tumors predominantly originate from the nasal mucosa near the middle meatus. They can invade the turbinates and remodel the nasal cavity, with displacement of the nasal septum and lateral bowing of the nasal wall. Hemangiomas are usually separated into capillary, cavernous or mixed hemangiomas. They are rare in

the paranasal sinuses and occur mainly in females between the ages of 20 and 50 years. They may complicate the second trimester of pregnancy, but regress spontaneously following the delivery (granuloma gravidarum). Hemangiomas enhance following the administration of intravenous contrast (Figure 9.11). On T1-weighted MR scans, they are intermediate in signal intensity; they are hyperintense on T2-weighted MR scans, with a surrounding rim of low signal intensity. Mucosal hemangiomas usually present with epistaxis and nasal obstruction. The osseous hemangiomas arise from the nasal septum or the nasal bones and tend to cause deformity. The surgical management is different for mucosal and osseous hemangiomas.

Angiofibroma

This rare condition usually affects male adolescents. The lesion arises from the medial pterygoid plate, the pterygomaxillary fissure and the sphenopalatine foramen, and not from the nasopharynx, where they usually present. The lesions are benign but, because they expand to involve the ethmoid sinuses, the sphenoid sinuses and the skull base, the clinical implications are sinister. It is important to determine whether there is intracranial extension of the angiofibroma via the orbital apex to the superior orbital fissure and thence to the middle cranial fossa. If this has occurred, it is usual for the lesion to obtain some of its blood supply from the internal carotid artery, and so surgical resection becomes more difficult and hazardous.

Radiologic features include enlargement of the sphenopalatine foramen, erosion of the medial pterygoid plate, widening of the pterygopalatine fossa and indentation of the posterior wall of the maxillary sinus. The nasopharyngeal mucosa may be thickened or irregular (Figure 9.12).

The angiofibroma is of homogenous density and strongly enhances following the administration of intravenous contrast. Angiography prior to embolization or excision will demonstrate the main feeding vessels.

INVERTING PAPILLOMAS

Most benign squamous papillomas occur on the septum or in the nasal vestibule. However, some types of papilloma do occur within the paranasal sinuses and may be seen as soft-tissue masses. These rarely cause bone erosion or undergo malignant transformation. One form of papilloma that does behave in a more sinister and aggressive manner is the inverting papilloma.

Inverting papillomas are uncommon neoplasms of the nasal cavity and paranasal sinuses. They occur more commonly in men than women, with the greatest incidence in the sixth and seventh decades. Inverting papillomas are slowly growing lesions that have a propensity to recur, especially if the initial excision is incomplete. There is much debate regarding the potential for malignant transformation of inverting papillomas. It is felt by many that the malignant tumor, when present, develops synchronously with the inverting papilloma and is present in the tissue resected at the initial operation. Others feel that the malignancy develops following transformation of the inverting papilloma. It is noteworthy that malignancy is rarely found after an initial resection in which excision was complete.

The clinical features include nasal obstruction, anosmia, rhinorrhea and epistaxis. Pain and facial paresthesia are not characteristic features of inverting papillomas, but they may be indicative of concurrent malignancy. Many of the patients have had multiple operations on the nose and paranasal sinuses prior to diagnosis. The most common site of origin is within the middle meatus, but extension into the adjacent sinus occurs frequently (Figure 9.13). The maxillary antrum is involved in 69% of cases followed by the ethmoid sinuses (Figures 9.14–9.16), sphenoid sinus (Figure 9.16), and the frontal sinus, in decreasing order of frequency. Inverting papilloma arising from the nasal septum are uncommon and bilateral disease is rare (Figure 9.17). Obstruction of the sinus ostia in the middle meatus may lead to the accumulation of secretions in the obstructed sinus and a secondary sinusitis. Rarely, one of the paranasal sinuses may be involved primarily, with no evidence of tumor extension into the nasal vault (Figure 9.16).

Plain radiographs are of limited value. One-third of plain radiographs are reported to be either normal or show nonspecific mucosal thickening. Other features noted on plain radiographs include opacity of the maxillary antrum, a soft-tissue mass in the nasal cavity, ethmoid opacification and frontal sinus disease. The bony walls of the paranasal sinuses and of the nasal vault may show remodeling, erosion, or reactive sclerosis.

CT can delineate bony erosion and clearly demonstrate the extent of the soft-tissue abnormalities (Figures 9.14 and 9.15). This is invaluable both in the preoperative assessment of these patients and in the long-term follow up that is required with inverting papillomas. The frequent finding of mucosal disease from concurrent allergic rhinitis or sinusitis may be misinterpreted as further extension of disease. The already noted high incidence of previous nasal surgery in these cases often distorts the radiographic features, making it more difficult to identify the limits of disease (Figures 9.17 and 9.18).

Sclerosis of the bony sinus walls has been noted in association with inverting papillomata, although this may well be related to an associated longstanding sinusitis rather than the papillomata. The radiologic appearance associated with an inverting papilloma is variable. If it is slow growing, the bony wall may be either thinned or eroded, and the opacity of the sinus will depend on the position and extent of the papilloma in relation to the ostia. Occasionally, areas of calcification will be demonstrated within the mass of the papilloma (Figure 9.18).

Tumor extension outside the confines of the nasal cavity and the paranasal sinuses is clearly demonstrated by CT. It is not uncommon to find tumor extending into the nasopharynx, usually in the form of a choanal polyp which may make contact with the posterior nasopharyngeal wall. The tumor may extend into the retrobulbar space causing exophthalmos, through the cribriform plate into the anterior cranial fossa, or through the greater wing of the sphenoid into the middle cranial fossa. On MR scans, these tumors exhibit low to intermediate signal intensity. The tumor itself can be separated from the surrounding inflammatory fluid in the obstructed sinus, as fluid is hyperintense on T2-weighted MR sequences.

MIDFACIAL NECROTIZING LESIONS

The midfacial destructive lesions have been given many names over the years. The two histologically distinct lesions described here, Wegener's granulomatosis and pleomorphic reticulosis, present in a similar manner but require radically different treatment.

Wegener's granulomatosis is a clinical diagnosis based upon the finding of systemic disease affecting the nasal cavity, kidneys and lung. It is characterized by a necrotizing granulomatous vasculitis.

Not uncommonly, there is associated orbital pathology, such as conjunctivitis, corneal–scleral ulceration, uveitis or optic neuritis. This may be the result of primary disease of the orbit, or the orbital symptoms may be related to spread of the disease from the paranasal sinuses. Treatment for Wegener's granulomatosis includes high-dose steroids and immunosuppressants.

The radiologic features of Wegener's granulomatosis (Figure 9.19) are nonspecific; the lesion appears on plain radiographs only as mucosal thickening with or without retained mucopus. Initially, the changes are similar to chronic inflammatory disease, with mucosal thickening in the sinonasal cavity. Subsequently, the nasal septum or the turbinates may be thickened or the granuloma may be seen as a soft-tissue mass on these structures. The final or the destructive stage is seen as irregular erosions of the septum. The turbinates may be destroyed, and the sinuses that are affected may be sclerotic, the sinus lumen being compromised by the fibro-osseous proliferation. In some cases, a secondary bacterial infection within the nose and paranasal sinuses is thought to account for the bony sclerosis that is often demonstrated by CT. Nonspecific irregular densities may be seen within the orbit which are associated with scleral–uveal thickening and muscle swelling.

The other main group in this category are pleomorphic reticulosis. This lesion behaves as a non-Hodgkin's (T cell) lymphoma, but the histologic diagnosis is difficult to reach in the early stages of the disease. The condition is treated with a combination of radiotherapy and chemotherapy. The radiologic features are of destruction of the soft tissue and bones of the midface. These changes are nonspecific and cannot be differentiated from granulomatous infection.

Rhinoliths

Many objects, both animate and inanimate, have been recovered from the nasal cavity. If a foreign body remains undisturbed for some time it will become covered in salts of calcium and magnesium. These are usually phosphates, oxalates and carbonates. Over a period of years the rhinolith can enlarge and become molded to the shape of the cavity in which it is situated. A rhinolith may present itself with nasal obstruction and a foul-smelling unilateral rhinorrhea. If large, the rhinolith will need to be disimpacted under general anesthetic.

The rhinolith is readily demonstrated on plain radiographs or CT as a radio-opaque lesion with sharply demarcated borders (Figure 9.20).

MALIGNANT TUMORS

Malignant tumors of the nose and paranasal sinuses are rare and account for 0.2–0.8% of all malignancies. Because of the concealed nature of the anatomy and the relative inocuity of the early symptoms, these tumors may often have reached an advanced stage prior to diagnosis. This and the morbidity associated with resection of the surrounding anatomic regions is responsible for their poor prognosis.

Initially, the symptoms may be similar to those of a chronic sinusitis with persistent rhinorrhea and facial pain. Progression of the symptoms to a persistent pain or paresthesia should warrant further investigation. Early evidence of bone erosion or asymmetrical sclerosis may be suggestive of an underlying malignancy.

The sinister symptoms associated with malignancy in the paranasal sinuses will depend upon the site of origin of the tumor. These may include facial pain and paresthesia, loosening of the teeth or a change in fit of a dental plate, exophthalmos, epiphora and nasal obstruction with a persistent discharge that may be blood stained. In the more advanced stages of the disease, the tumor often involves more than one sinus.

The commonest site of malignancy in the paranasal sinuses is the maxillary antrum, where the majority of malignant tumors arise. The second most common site is the ethmoid sinus. It is rare for tumors to arise in either the frontal or the sphenoid sinuses.

The commonest tumor in the paranasal sinuses is squamous cell carcinoma, followed by undifferentiated carcinoma, adenoid cystic carcinoma and adenocarcinoma. Other tumors occur infrequently and include malignant lymphoma, malignant melanoma, esthesioneuroblastoma, plasmocytoma, metastatic tumors and the sarcomas.

The diagnosis of paranasal sinus malignancy requires an accurate history and a thorough clinical examination, including endoscopic examination. Plain radiography and conventional tomography have a minor role in diagnosis but have been superceded by CT and MR. These last two modalities have a very important role in identifying features

Table 9.1   The TNM classification of tumors of the maxillary sinus.

T1   Tumors are confined to the antral mucosa of the anteroinferior portion, without bone erosion or destruction

T2   Tumors are confined to the posterosuperior portion, without bone erosion, or to the anteroinferior portion, with erosion of the medial or inferior bony walls

T3   Tumors invade the skin, orbits, anterior ethmoid sinuses or the pterygoid muscles

T4   Tumors invade the cribriform plate, posterior ethmoid sinuses, sphenoid sinuses, pterygoid plates, nasopharynx or skull base

N0   No clinically positive nodes

N1   a single clinically positive, ipsilateral lymph node <3 cm in diameter

N2   a single clinically positive, ipsilateral lymph node, 6–3 cm in diameter, or multiple ipsilateral nodes <6 cm in diameter

N3   massive ipsilateral nodes, bilateral nodes or a contralateral node

M0   no distant metastases

M1   distant metastases present

depending upon their position relative to Ohngren's line. This is a plane extending from the medial canthus of the eye to the angle of the mandible, dividing the maxillary antrum into an anteroinferior and a posterosuperior portion.

Imaging plays an important role in the management of patients with malignancies in the sinuses or nasopharynx. Both MR and CT are used to define the margins and extent of the tumor, and for the assessment of any involvement of the vital structures such as the cranial nerves, the orbit and the intracranial structures. Postoperative and postradiation follow up is best done with these two modalities. Neither MR nor CT can distinguish between the various histologic types of malignancy.

Plain radiography

Plain radiographs are often the initial radiologic investigation requested for a patient with sinus symptoms that are refractory to medical treatment. The bony margins should be examined for asymmetry and/or bony destruction. The margins of particular interest are the medial wall of the antrum and the orbit, the ethmomaxillary plate, the infraorbital foramen and the skull base. Clouding and opacification of the sinuses are common to both inflammatory and malignant lesions. Erosions where the bone is normally thin along the medial wall of the maxillary sinus, the lamina papyracea and the infraorbital groove is often accompanied with reactive osteitis in benign inflammatory diseases. Destruction due to malignancy is seen to involve the posterior and inferolateral walls of the maxilla, and tumors do not usually evoke new bone formation.

suggestive of malignancy and in the staging of the lesion. The final pathologic diagnosis follows tissue biopsy and histologic examination.

Tumors arising in the maxillary sinus are staged according to the TNM classification (Table 9.1). The TNM staging is used by radiotherapists, oncologists and surgeons to decide which will be the most appropriate form of treatment for the patient and to compare the long-term results of different treatment modalities. As yet there are no adequate staging protocols for malignancy of the frontal, ethmoid or sphenoid sinuses. The maxillary sinuses are staged

Computed Tomography

Computed tomography is the imaging modality of choice for the assessment of the bony margins and soft-tissue extension of a malignancy of the paranasal sinuses. Indications for CT are given in Table 9.2.

Usually the scans are conducted in both the axial and the coronal planes at 5 mm intervals following the administration of a bolus of intravenous contrast. It is important to scan the whole sinus and surrounding soft-tissue area to identify any tumor that has escaped from the sinus cavity.

Table **9.2** Indications for CT of benign tumors.

The symptoms of rhinosinusitis persist for more than 2 months despite aggressive antibiotic treatment

Suspicious clinical features occur, such as paresthesia, palpable mass or blood-stained rhinorrhea

Plain radiographs demonstrate suspicious areas of bone erosion

To assess the extent and to stage a tumor prior to planning treatment

In the axial plane, CT is useful for demonstrating the posterior extension of tumors of the maxilla into the pterygopalatine fossa, the infratemporal fossa and the soft tissue of the cheek (Figures 9.21 and 9.22). The coronal plane is superior to the axial for demonstrating intraorbital and frontal sinus involvement as well as spread through the cribriform plate or planum sphenoidale into the anterior cranial fossa (Figure 9.23).

The administration of intravenous contrast demonstrates a variable pattern of enhancement. The result depends mainly upon the vascularity of the tumor, for example, the hemangiosarcomas, metastatic hypernephroma, esthesioneuroblastoma and some rhabdomyosarcomas enhance more vigorously than other tumors. The pattern of enhancement is also influenced by the presence of retained secretions or chronic infection within a sinus; this will appear as an area of reduced enhancement (Figure 9.25). Similarly, necrotic centres of tumor masses also enhance less and have a lower density than the surrounding tumor which tends to be isodense with muscle. The administration of contrast also helps to identify the surrounding blood vessels and their relationship to the tumor mass.

The clarity with which CT demonstrates the soft tissue and the bony architecture of the paranasal sinuses is of great value in assessing the presence of malignancy within a sinus. The soft tissue within the sinus in question may exhibit irregular margins and the mucosa may be considerably thickened. This mucosal thickening may be due to an inflammatory reaction surrounding the tumor or due to tumor invasion itself (Figures 9.24 and 9.26). It is not possible to distinguish which of these processes is responsible using the imaging technique.

Most malignant tumors of the paranasal sinuses have an homogenous appearance. The exceptions are the minor salivary gland tumors and the schwannomas, which exhibit a nonhomogenous pattern. Areas of retained secretions and necrosis may be demonstrated, as already discussed.

Bony remodeling or new bone formation is rarely seen with tumors of the paranasal sinuses, with the exception of ossifying osteosarcomas. However, malignant tumors often arise in sinuses that have been the site of chronic inflammation; consequently, the bony changes may reflect this previous disease. Calcified deposits occur within the tumor masses of fibroosseous lesions, chondrosarcoma and the osteosarcomas. With most tumors the bone is thinned or eroded in an irregular manner (Figure 9.21). If the sinus is expanded and has an intact but thinned bony wall, then it is more likely that the lesion is benign. The absence of bone destruction does not exclude the possibility of an early malignant lesion, and biopsy should be performed if clinically indicated. However, the presence of a slowly growing tumor cannot be eliminated. Aggressive bone destruction of the sinus walls is usually suggestive of a squamous cell carcinoma, but it may also represent a metastatic deposit from a distant primary site such as lung, breast, kidney or gastrointestinal tract. Radioisotope bone scans are sensitive for bony metastases. If a sinonasal lesion is suspected to be of metastatic origin, then a bone scan will establish the secondary nature of the lesion if multiple bones are involved. Local invasion from tumors arising in the adjacent structures are not uncommon. When such invasion involves the entire sinus, it is difficult to be sure of the exact site of origin.

Further evidence that a tumor has escaped primarily from the confines of the sinus involved is gained from a careful examination of the fat planes lying between the soft tissue of the surrounding areas. These planes are usually well demonstrated by CT, and obliteration or distortion of them is suggestive of either edema, hemorrhage or tumor infiltration. When advanced, tumors of the paranasal sinuses may involve more than one sinus and the primary site may be obscured by widespread destruction. Likewise, it may be difficult to differentiate the site of origin of a tumor if the nasopharynx, sphenoid and/or the pituitary fossa are involved (Figures 9.22 and 9.27). A tumor arising in the paranasal sinuses readily escapes into the pterygopalatine fossa (Figure 9.21 and 9.22), the infratemporal fossa, the orbital apex (Figure 9.28), the orbital cavity (Figure 9.29), the middle cranial fossa, and the nasopharynx. Tumors may also spread through the many foramina in the skull base that transmit nerves and vessels into the orbit and face, thus gaining easy access to the anterior and middle cranial fossa.

If lymph-node metastases is suspected clinically, CT can demonstrate enlarged nodes in the submandibular lateral retropharyngeal space and in the upper deep cervical lymph nodes. These nodes are usually the first to become involved, with metastatic spread through the lymphatic system secondary to malignancy in the paranasal sinuses. Imaging is the ideal way to assess nodal metastases, as physical examination will not identify small lymph nodes in the deep spaces of the neck.

CT has a valuable role in the follow up of patients who have been treated for a malignancy of the paranasal sinuses. It is important to obtain a baseline scan about 6 weeks following surgery to delineate the boundaries of the surgical defect. By this time most of the soft-tissue irregularities that follow as a result of the surgery will have settled and the margins of the cavity should be smooth. Repeat scans should then be obtained every 3–6 months to try to detect any tumor recurrence as early as is possible, before salvage surgery becomes impossible.

Signs suggestive of recurrent tumor include soft-tissue expansion, especially of a polypoid nature. This may only represent fibrous scarring of the mucosa, but it will direct the surgeon to the site(s) requiring biopsy. Either thickening or further destruction of the remaining bones of the cavity are also sinister findings that warrant further investigation. Care should be taken to differentiate the bone dehiscence secondary to the surgical defect and that which may be secondary to tumor recurrence. The presence of an expanded mass on the image is suggestive of advanced recurrent disease.

If the patient has been treated with radiotherapy, chemotherapy or a combination of both, CT should demonstrate tumor regression; again, a baseline scan taken after the treatment response has subsided will be of value in following the patient's clinical progress. There is usually an acute inflammatory response that enhances clearly in the initial phase of treatment, but this has usually subsided 6–8 weeks following completion of treatment. Difficulties arise in the assessment of the images of patients who have developed extensive scar tissue as a consequence of both the tumor and the surgical and/or radiotherapeutic treatment. In these patients, it is often impossible to differentiate scar tissue from recurrent tumor without biopsy. Nodularity of the mucosa is more in keeping with tumor recurrence. Follow-up scans should be done at 3 month, 6 month and yearly intervals.

It is not possible to make a sound diagnosis of the histologic type of the tumor from radiographic findings alone, and biopsy is mandatory. Certain features, however, may be suggestive of the type of tumor. Aggressive bone erosion is usually caused by squamous cell carcinoma, lymphoepitheliomas and lymphomas. These tumors may also contain calcified fragments.

The mucoepidermoid and adenocarcinomas tend to be slow growing, and initially the sinus may appear expanded. If untreated, bone destruction will occur. These masses must be differentiated from metastatic deposits from lung, breast and the renal tract.

The olfactory neuroblastoma or esthesioneuroblastoma arises from cells of neural crest origin within the olfactory mucosa; it may extend into the ethmoid and sphenoid sinuses, as well as intracranially (Figure 9.23). The tumor is slow growing, vascular and friable, and enhances following the administration of intravenous contrast.

Chondrosarcomas, osteosarcomas and other tumors of cartilaginous or osseous origin often exhibit areas of calcification within an expanded sinus. The histologic diagnosis may be suggested by this appearance.

Angiography is not routinely done in the evaluation of sinonasal tumors. Angiofibromas, sarcomas and some vascular metastases exhibit intense vascularity. If embolization of the tumor prior to debulking the tumor mass is to be done, then angiography is undertaken.

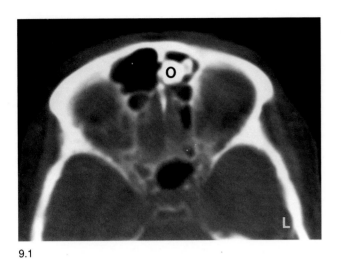

9.1

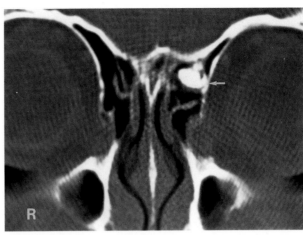

9.2

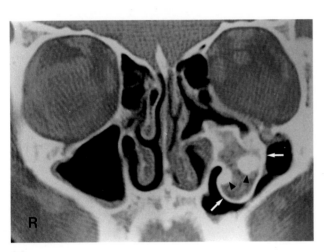

9.3

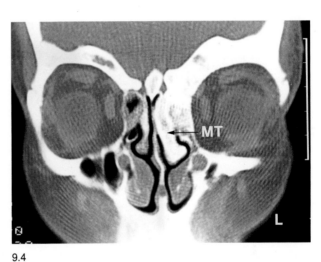

9.4

Figure **9.1**

Frontal sinus osteoma: CT scan. The dense bony mass (O) seen in the frontal sinus is an osteoma.

Figure **9.2**

Frontal recess osteoma. This CT scan demonstrates a well-defined bony mass in the anterior ethmoid air cells without bony destruction. This is the characteristic appearance of a benign osteoma (arrow). If large, the osteoma may occlude the sinus ostium, although on most occasions it is an incidental finding.

Figure **9.3**

Ossifying fibroma. This CT scan demonstrates an unusual mass in the left maxillary sinus. This has the radiologic features of an ossifying fibroma. Note the sclerotic margins of the mass (arrows) and the ovoid areas of calcification (arrowheads) within the mass.

Figure **9.4**

Fibrous dysplasia. This CT scan demonstrates thickening of the orbital roof and the superomedial aspect of the orbit. The entire left middle turbinate (MT) is thickened and replaced by abnormal bone.

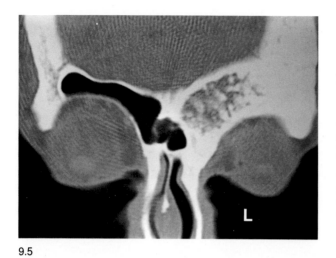

9.5

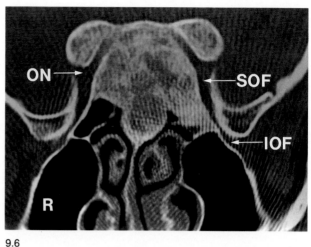

9.6

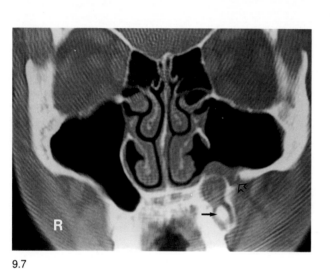

9.7

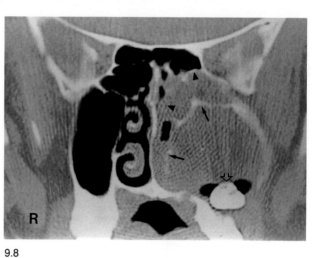

9.8

Figure 9.5

Fibrous dysplasia. This wide-window coronal CT scan demonstrates the characteristic 'ground-glass' appearance of fibrous dysplasia affecting the left frontal bone. If the sinuses are viewed with a narrow window, then this abnormality could be mistaken for inflammatory disease in the left frontal sinus.

Figure 9.6

Fibrous dysplasia: CT scan. The entire sphenoid bone is thickened with the typical ground glass appearance of fibrous dysplasia. The superior orbital fissure (SOF), the optic nerve canal (ON) and the inferior orbital fissure (IOF) are demonstrated.

Figure 9.7

Odentogenic keratocyst. This coronal CT scan demonstrates a cystic lesion in the left alveolar ridge; it has a smooth scalloped margin. The unerupted tooth can be seen in the base of the cyst (arrow). The defect in the anterior bony wall of the maxilla (open arrow) is evidence of a previous Caldwell–Luc procedure. Incomplete resection results in recurrence. These cysts can be multiloculated.

Figure 9.8

Dentigerous cyst: CT scan. A large expansile cyst (arrow) is demonstrated containing an unerupted tooth (open arrow). The maxillary sinus walls are remodelled and the inferolateral wall of the maxillary sinus is eroded. The sinus is extending medially into the nasal cavity (arrowheads).

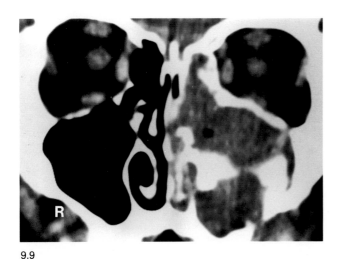

9.9

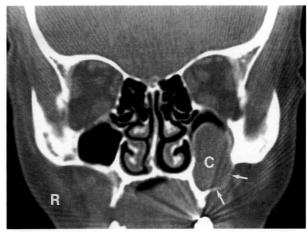

9.10

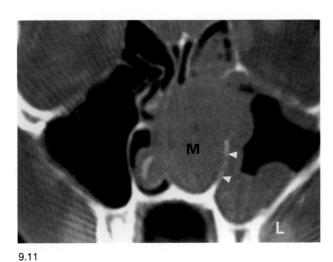

9.11

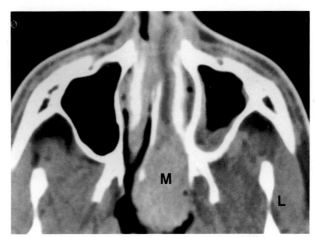

9.12

Figure **9.9**

Dentigerous cyst. This CT scan taken with a narrow setting shows the cyst and the maxillary sinus are filled with fluid of a uniform density.

Figure **9.11**

Hemangioma. This CT scan demonstrates a soft-tissue mass (M) in the left nasal cavity. As a result of the chronic exertion of pressure on the bone, there has been smooth expansion of the nasal cavity with marked lateral bowing of the lateral wall of the nose (arrows). The ostiomeatal complex is occluded by this large mass and there is a polypoid configuration of the mucosa in the left maxillary sinus. This was proved to be a benign hemangioma, but there are no specific radiologic characteristics that can point to the diagnosis.

Figure **9.10**

Dentigerous cyst. This coronal CT scan demonstrates an expansile cyst (C) with a bony rim arising in the floor of the right maxillary sinus. This was a large pyogenic, dentigerous cyst. The tooth to which it was related is not demonstrated in these scans. Note the erosion and thinning of the maxillary sinus wall (arrows). This is one of the few occasions when inflammation of the sinus is found in conjunction with a normal ostiomeatal complex, and where treatment must be directed at the lesion itself.

Figure **9.12**

Angiofibroma. This axial CT scan demonstrates a soft-tissue mass (M), in the left nasal cavity. It has caused widening of the left posterior choana and the nasal septum is deviated to the right. There is mucosal thickening in the left maxillary sinus. This was found to be an angiofibroma.

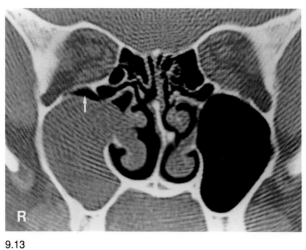

9.13

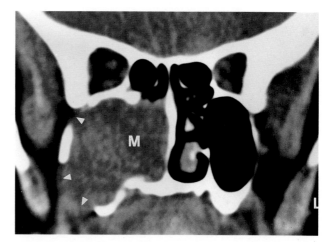

9.14A

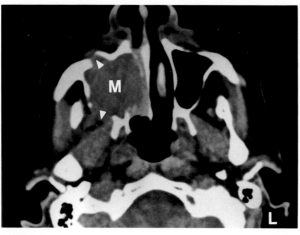

9.14B

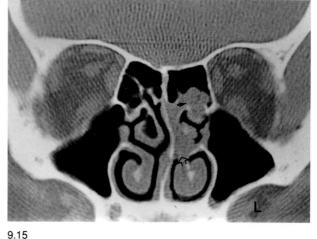

9.15

Figure **9.13**

Inverting papilloma. This CT scan demonstrates a well-defined soft-tissue mass with a meniscus of air in the maxillary sinus. The mass is seen protruding into the posterior part of the middle meatus. There is no calcification in the mass and there are areas of reactive new bone formation. There are no radiologic features of this mass to distinguish it from an antrochoanal polyp. A meniscus of air above the mass (arrow) is more a feature of polypoid disease rather than a mucocele.

Figure **9.14**

Inverting papilloma. Both the coronal (A) and axial (B) CT scans demonstrate a smooth expansile mass (M) in the right maxillary sinus. There is erosion of the anterior, posterior, medial and inferolateral walls of the sinus (arrowheads). In benign disease of the paranasal sinuses, bony erosion occurs in close proximity to the natural ostia, i.e. near the infraorbital foramen and the medial sinus wall. In this case, the erosion has occurred in atypical sites and the radiologist should be suspicious that this is not a benign polyp.

Figure **9.15**

Inverting papilloma. This coronal CT of the paranasal sinuses demonstrates a unilateral soft-tissue mass (arrow) arising from the superior meatus, extending from above the horizontal plate of the middle turbinate medially into the nasal cavity just alongside the free margin of the middle turbinate. The mass is in close proximity to the inferior turbinate on the left side (open arrow). The middle meatus appears normal. There is no evidence of erosion of the underlying bones. Clinically this was proved to be an inverting papilloma arising from the posterior ethmoid air cells and the superior meatus.

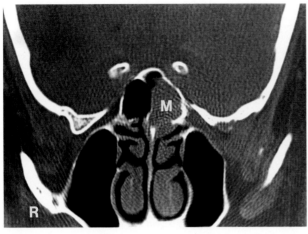

9.16A

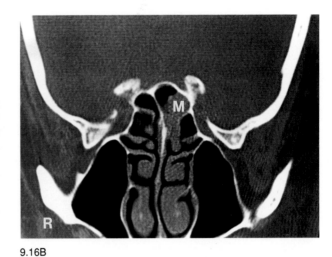

9.16B

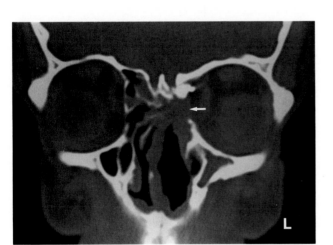

9.17A

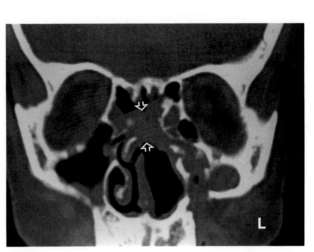

9.17B

Figure **9.16**

Inverting papilloma: CT scans. One of the unusual presenting sites for an inverting papilloma is the sphenoid sinus. The mass (M) which arose in the left sphenoid sinus, has caused erosion of the floor of that sphenoid sinus and can be seen protruding into the sphenoethmoidal recess. There is reactive bony sclerosis of the lateral wall of the left sphenoid sinus. Note in (B) how the tumor has extended into the superior meatus.

Figure **9.17**

Inverting papilloma: CT scans. Postoperative views of the sinuses demonstrate a defect in the lamina papyracea from a previous external ethmoidectomy (arrow) with removal of the ethmomaxillary plate. There is soft-tissue proliferation, extending to involve the nasal septum and the opposite ethmoid sinuses (open arrows). This patient had a recurrent inverting papilloma. It is unusual for the papilloma to involve both nasal cavities, The bony septa in the ethmoid air cells indicate that the previous ethmoidectomy was incomplete.

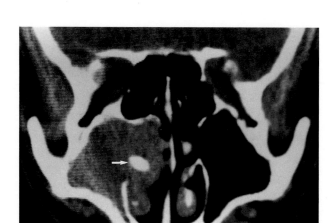

9.18

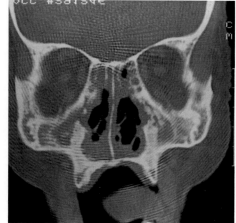

9.19

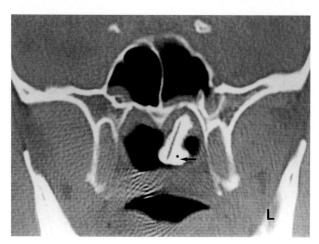
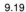

9.20

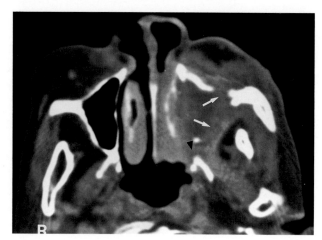

9.21

Figure **9.18**

Inverting papilloma. This coronal CT scan demonstrates large nodular calcification (arrow) in an expansile mass involving the middle meatus and right maxillary sinus. This was an inverting papilloma.

Figure **9.19**

Wegener's granulomatosis. This coronal CT scan demonstrates destruction of the turbinates, with an excessive amount of inflammatory reaction and reactive osteitis.

Figure **9.20**

Rhinolith. This patient presented with a long history of halitosis and a mass was seen in the nasopharynx on clinical examination. The CT scan shows a rhinolith in the nose which has formed around a tiddlywink. This has caused extensive inflammatory reaction and the rhinolith (arrow) was seen molding around the inferior turbinate and into the nasopharynx.

Figure **9.21**

Carcinoma of the floor of the mouth involving the maxillary sinus. This patient presented with an ulcer on the left cheek. She was a betal-nut chewer. On CT, a mass is seen eroding the hard plate and the floor of the nasal cavity and extending into the maxillary sinus. Note the fluid in the left maxillary sinus and the destruction of the sinus walls (arrows). There is faint irregular enhancement of the sinus mucosa, indicating tumor invasion. The pterygopalatine fossa is involved posteriorly (arrowhead).

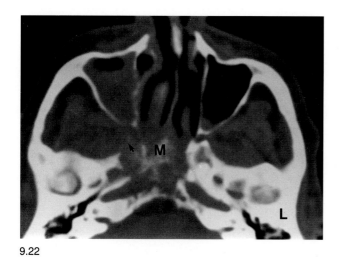

9.22

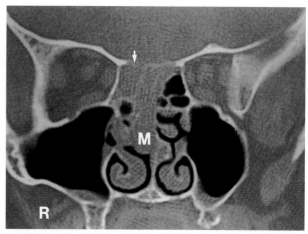

9.23

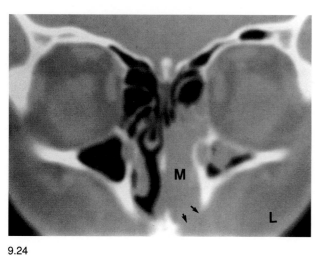

9.24

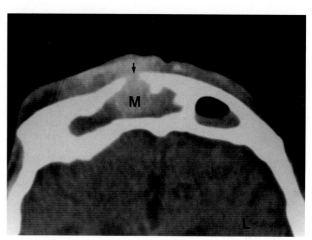

9.25

Figure **9.22**

Nasopharyngeal carcinoma. This patient presented with a history of sinusitis that was refractory to medical treatment. A mass (M) destroying the base of the skull is seen on this CT. The right maxillary sinusitis can be seen as well as destruction of the pterygoid plates and the posterior wall of the maxillary sinus (arrow) following invasion of the pterygopalatine fossa.

Figure **9.23**

Esthesioneuroblastoma. A soft-tissue mass is seen on this CT in the roof of the nasal cavity with destruction of the roof of the ethmoid (arrow). The mass (M) extends into the superior meatus, medial to the middle turbinate.

Figure **9.24**

Non-Hodgkin's lymphoma. This coronal CT scan demonstrates a soft-tissue mass (M), filling the left nasal cavity and middle meatus. The bone of the floor of the left nasal cavity has been eroded (arrows).

Figure **9.25**

Non-Hodgkin's lymphoma. This axial CT scan, following the administration of contrast, demonstrates an enhancing mass (M) in the frontal sinus which is surrounded by fluid of lower density. There is destruction of the anterior wall of the frontal sinus (arrow).

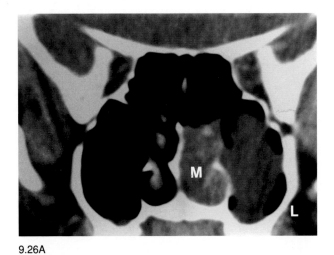

9.26A

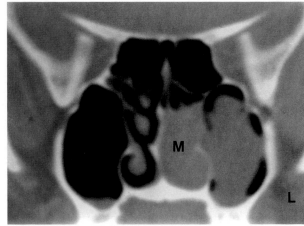

9.26B

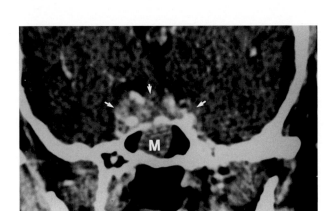

9.27A

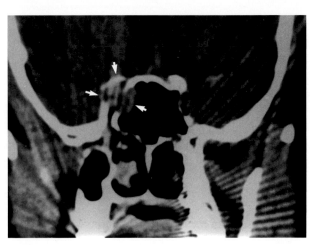

9.27B

Figure **9.26**

Non-Hodgkin's lymphoma. These narrow- (A) and wide-window (B) coronal CT scans are of the same patient in Figure 9.24. The soft-tissue mass (M), can be seen extending posteriorly throughout the left nasal cavity. In the narrow-window scan the soft tissue within the left maxillary sinus appears less dense than the mass in the left nasal cavity and reflects retained secretions.

Figure **9.27**

Pituitary tumor. These coronal CT scans demonstrate an enhancing mass that has eroded through the floor of the pituitary fossa and extended inferiorly into the sphenoid sinus (M) and laterally to involve the internal carotid artery, optic nerve and superior part of the superior orbital fissure. This was a benign functioning chromophobe adenoma (arrows).

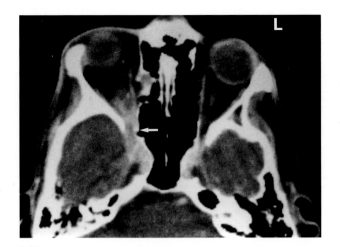

9.28

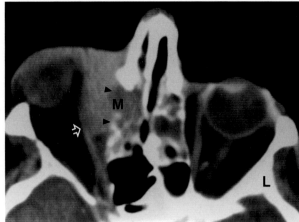

9.29

Figure **9.28**

Tumor extension through the superior orbital fissure. This axial CT scan demonstrates extension of tumor through the right superior orbital fissure (arrow), into the orbit.

Figure **9.29**

Non-Hodgkin's lymphoma. This axial CT scan shows tumor (M) extending from the ethmoid sinus into the orbit. The lamina papyracea has been eroded (arrowheads). The intraorbital extension has deviated the medial rectus muscle (open arrow) laterally and the eyeball is exophthalmos. This was subsequently diagnosed as a non-Hodgkin's lymphoma.

10

The postoperative appearances of the paranasal sinuses

It is important for the radiologist to have a working knowledge of the indications for sinus surgery and of the variety of surgical approaches that are used, as well as the surgical complications that may result from these procedures. The bony defects and some of the soft-tissue abnormalities created by the different surgical approaches are discussed in this chapter so that the incorrect interpretation of surgical bony defects as bone erosion can be avoided. Comparison with the preoperative scans will also help eliminate this potential source of error. It is important for the radiologist to understand the reasons why the surgeon will on occasion request postoperative computed tomography (CT). A postoperative CT is usually done 6–8 weeks after surgery in those problem cases where there is a persistence of symptoms. These may include the identification of the reason for an unsuccessful procedure, such as missed disease, of scarring of the areas critical for ventilation and drainage or simply of recurrent disease which may require revision surgery. In addition, it is important for the surgeon to be aware of potential danger areas, for example, a previously unrecognized breech of the lamina papyracea or of the cribriform plate.

Plain radiographs are inadequate for the assessment of a patient with recurrent paranasal sinusitis following surgery because, in these cases, recurrent disease and postoperative fibrosis will appear simply to be increased opacification. It is well documented that CT and magnetic resonance imaging (MR) are the two most reliable methods for the assessment of paranasal sinus disease. CT has two important roles in the management of those patients who have undergone previous sinus surgery. The first is to indicate where residual or recurrent disease is located if the patient either remains symptomatic or develops a recurrence of symptoms. Clinical evaluation alone is inadequate to assess the site off failure, and accurate radiological assessment increases the chances of identifying and subsequently eradicating the disease. When recurrence of

malignancy is suspected, MR is far superior to CT because with MR the signal intensity of tumor recurrence is different from scar tissue and might direct the surgeon to suspicious areas for biopsy.

Surgery conducted for the excision of an inverting papilloma or a malignancy demands accurate follow up. These patients should have CT or MR scans at 3–6 month intervals; the scans are compared to the initial baseline postoperative scan. This process will identify those changes that represent recurrent disease. Following the administration of intravenous contrast, inflammatory tissue can usually be differentiated from scar tissue or mucocele, although this is not infallible, and adequate clinical information must be provided to help in the interpretation of the postoperative CT and MR scans.

The second role of computed tomography is in the preoperative assessment of patients requiring revision sinus surgery. The images will enable the identification of the extent of the previous surgery, any anatomic changes that may have occurred as a consequence of the procedure and the sites of residual disease. Postoperative changes include scarring, fibrosis, synechia and bony sclerosis. The sclerotic changes are usually at the expense of the interior of the sinus, resulting in a small sinus cavity with dense, thickened walls (Figures 10.14, 10.15 and 10.23).

Surgery may fail to eradicate benign inflammatory disease of the paranasal sinuses for a variety of reasons. In our experience, the commonest cause of failure is incomplete marsupialization of the ethmoid air cells, especially those of the anterior ethmoid or agger nasi. This is especially common following intranasal ethmoidectomy, and the residual bony septa are seen with soft-tissue abnormalities. These residual bony septa are best demonstrated on CT (Figures 10.17 and 10.18). Atopic individuals are more prone to recurrent disease with hyperplastic rhinosinusitis. Occasionally, recurrent maxillary sinus disease will occur despite the absence of disease in the ostiomeatal complex or nasal cavity. This is difficult to explain but may be related to disordered ciliary motility.

In this chapter, we give brief descriptions of the indications, surgical technique and related radiographic features of the more frequently performed sinus procedures, followed by a discussion of the radiologic appearances of complications of surgery.

INFERIOR MEATAL ANTROSTOMY

In inferior meatal antrostomy, also called an inferior antral window, drainage is facilitated through an opening in the dependent part of the maxillary sinus. This procedure has fallen out of favor as the mucociliary beat mechanism is always directed toward the natural ostium of the maxillary sinus.

Indication

Chronic maxillary sinusitis and biopsy of soft-tissue masses within the maxillary antrum.

Technique

The inferior turbinate is retracted medially. The lateral wall of the inferior meatus is perforated and, if necessary, the surrounding bone is excised. The antrostomy is extended down to the floor of the nasal cavity and anteroposteriorly to a diameter of 1.5–2.0 cm. Some surgeons resect all or part of the inferior turbinate to facilitate antroscopy at a later date.

Radiologic features

The bony defect is evident in the inferior meatus. With time, this may stenose, with either bony or mucosal regeneration (Figures 10.1–10.3). If the patient continues to be symptomatic following this conventional procedure, then obstruction to the ostiomeatal complex is probably present.

CALDWELL–LUC PROCEDURE

This is one of the oldest surgical procedures used to treat chronic maxillary sinusitis.

Indications

Chronic maxillary sinusitis, removal of dental roots, excision of antrochoanal polyps, tumors, mucoceles, odontogenic or denteriginous cysts and repair of oroantral fistulae. To access the orbital floor for decompression surgery, for elevation of the orbital floor for the reduction of fractures and for access to the pterygopalatine fossa either for ligation of the internal maxillary artery for uncontrolled epistaxis or for a pterygoid (vidian) neurectomy in patients with intractable vasomotor rhinitis.

Technique

A sublabial approach is made through the anterior wall of the maxillary sinus via the canine fossa. This is situated superolateral to the root of the upper canine teeth and inferior to the infraorbital nerve; it provides wide exposure and access to the maxillary sinus. The sublabial antrostomy is sometimes referred to as a radical antrostomy. If the indication for the surgery is chronic sinusitis or an antrochoanal polyp, the mucosa is then stripped from the entire antrum. If the indication for the procedure is to provide access to the pterygopalatine fossa the mucosa is left intact. An inferior meatal antrostomy is fashioned as described previously to facilitate drainage and to allow inspection of the antrum. It should be of sufficient proportion to prevent stenosis.

Radiologic features

Both plain radiography and CT are valuable prior to a Caldwell–Luc procedure (Figures 10.3 and 10.4). If plain radiography fails to demonstrate a normal volume maxillary sinus, CT will be necessary to exclude a hypoplastic maxillary sinus, which may be a contraindication to the surgery. A septated maxillary sinus may also be missed, leading to incomplete surgical drainage of both compartments. A Caldwell-Luc procedure through a hypoplastic sinus could result in dangerous complications such as perforation of the floor of the orbit and intraorbital soft tissue injury.

Clinical and radiographic improvement occurs in about 68% of patients undergoing this form of sinus surgery. However, one should avoid routine postoperative radiographic examinations in the first 6–8 weeks, as the presence of blood and edematous tissue may appear radiologically similar to disease. It is common to find an air–fluid level in the first few weeks following surgery and this may be misinterpreted as acute maxillary sinusitis. In assessing the postoperative images, the radiologist needs to differentiate between those changes that have occurred as a consequence of the surgical procedure and those abnormalities that may reflect continuing or recurrent disease. The clinical history is of great importance as some patients will still exhibit radiologic evidence of disease but may in fact be asymptomatic. Excessive soft-tissue proliferation in the sinonasal cavity could be polyps, loculated fluid or scarring, and without clinical information it can be misdiagnosed as tumor, especially if bony septa have been surgically removed.

Normal aeration of the maxillary sinuses occurs in approximately 20% of maxillary antra postoperatively and certainly the antrum may be partially aerated in a much greater proportion. Certain chronic changes have been noted to occur in the maxillary sinus following surgery. These are, in order of decreasing frequency, fibro-osseous proliferation, antral contraction and compartmentalization (Figures 10.4 and 10.14).

Fibro-osseous proliferation is thought to be secondary to both the resorption of blood and epithelium as well as the degree of re-epithelialization. New bone formation has also been noted in this area following trauma, although the mechanism of this bony proliferation is unclear and the process uncommon. Fibro-osseous proliferation will be shown by opacification of the maxillary antrum on plain radiographs, but only CT is able to accurately differentiate between bone and soft tissue (Figures 10.14 and 10.18).

The second abnormality noted is antral contraction. This may be associated with depression of the orbital floor, lateralization of the lateral nasal wall with consequent enlargement of the ipsilateral nasal cavity and is accompanied by fibro-osseous proliferation (Figure 10.5).

The third, and most uncommon, abnormality is compartmentalization. This is considered to be due to an altered tissue response during the healing process (Figure 10.4).

Bony irregularities resulting from the inferior meatal antrostomy and the sublabial antrostomy may be seen. The sublabial antrostomy usually closes with fibrous tissue or new bone formation, although it may persist in rare cases as an oroantral fistula.

Recurrent disease in the maxillary antrum following a Caldwell–Luc procedure may be difficult to identify radiologically, especially in the presence of fibrosis of the antrum (Figures 10.3 and 10.4). Total opacity of the antrum when previously it had been noted to be partially or wholly aerated, or an air–fluid level are both positive findings. Complications following a Caldwell–Luc procedure are uncommon, although osteomyelitis and osteoma formation have been reported. The immediate complications could be injury to the floor of the orbit, the optic nerve or the globe (Figures 10.33–10.36).

A more frequent late complication is that of mucocele formation that may occur many years following surgery. Mucocele formation is radiologically associated with a homogenous opacification of the maxillary sinus, erosion of the bony margins of the antrum and, occasionally dehiscence of the antral walls. There are two types of mucocele: primary and secondary. Primary mucoceles are the most common, and occur following the obstruction of the sinus ostium and occupy the whole sinus cavity. Secondary mucoceles are usually laterally placed with an aerated antrum medially.

ETHMOIDECTOMY

The surgical approaches to the ethmoid sinuses are many and varied. A brief description of the more commonly performed procedures follows. The radiologic features are similar in each case, with variations in the bony defects dependent on the approach used. The radiographic features are summarized together.

Transnasal ethmoidectomy

Transnasal ethmoidectomy

Indication

Multiple ethmoidal polyps.

Technique

Traditionally this procedure is carried out with the operative field being viewed directly through a speculum. The middle turbinate is retracted medially, thereby exposing the uncinate process and the ethmoid bulla. The bulla is opened and removed, allowing further dissection of the ethmoid labyrinth and excision of diseased mucosa. This is easier posteriorly, and the posterior ethmoid air cells and the sphenoid may be exposed. It is difficult to open the anterior or agger nasi cells by this approach (Figure 10.6).

Intranasal ethmoidectomy is more controlled if conducted endoscopically; this will be discussed later.

Transantral ethmoidectomy

Indications

Chronic maxillary and ethmoid sinusitis, orbital decompression.

Technique

This procedure was described by Jansen and Horgan and combines a Caldwell–Luc procedure with partial clearance of the ethmoid labyrinth. The Caldwell–Luc sublabial antrostomy is conducted as previously described. Forceps are then directed upwards and medially through the ethmomaxillary plate located in the superomedial angle of the maxillary sinus, being angled towards the contralateral parietal eminence. This opening into the posterior ethmoid air cells is then enlarged and the accessible cells cleared (Figure 10.7). It is not possible to adequately clear the anterior cells using this procedure.

External ethmoidectomy

Indications

Chronic ethmoid sinusitis, recurrent inflammatory nasal polyps, approach to the pituitary fossa.

Technique

This operation was first described by Ferris Smith in 1933. A temporary tarsorrhaphy is performed to protect the cornea. A curved incision is then made in the nasofacial fold onto the nasal bones, and the periosteum and lacrimal sac elevated. The orbital periosteum is then elevated to expose the anterior ethmoid artery and the contents of the orbit are retracted laterally. The anterior ethmoid artery is

then divided and the lamina papyracea is perforated, thereby opening the ethmoid air cells. The bony leaflets dividing the air cells are excised and the middle turbinate then visualized. Access may be gained as far posteriorly as the sphenoid sinus.

Transorbital ethmoidectomy

Indications

Orbital decompression, orbital trauma.

Technique

This technique was described by Patterson. The incision is placed 1 cm below the infraorbital margin. The orbicularis oculi muscle is divided by the periosteum. The periosteum is then elevated off the floor of the orbit and the lacrimal fossa, taking care not to damage the origin of the inferior oblique muscle or the nasolacrimal duct. The lamina papyracea is removed superiorly to the level of the frontoethmoid suture, and the floor of the orbit is removed as far laterally as the infraorbital canal. The frontal and sphenoid sinuses may be entered using this approach.

Functional endoscopic sinus surgery

Current thinking has focused surgery on the ventilation and drainage channels that serve the larger paranasal sinuses, especially the frontal and the maxillary sinuses. The removal of disease from the fine clefts of the ethmoid complex into which these channels connect allows normal ventilation of the paranasal sinuses and the reversal of mucosal disease within the larger sinuses to return to normal.

The degree to which the middle meatus can be examined has increased dramatically with the advent of CT and rigid endoscopy. It is now possible to accurately identify the sites of mucosal disease and anatomic variations that impede the ventilation and drainage channels, and to resect these areas using a focused and precisely targeted minimally invasive surgical approach (Figures 10.8 and 10.9).

Indications

Chronic sinusitis, recurrent inflammatory nasal polyposis, frontal and maxillary sinus mucoceles, biopsy decompression of a subperiosteal abscess.

Technique

Following adequate vasoconstriction an incision is made in the lateral wall of the nose, parallel to the free margin of the uncinate process. This bony leaflet is then elevated and excised, exposing the ethmoid bulla and the depths of the ethmoid infundibulum. It should now be possible to visualize the natural ostium of the maxillary sinus and that of the frontal recess. Further mucosal disease may then be removed under direct vision, to ensure both passages are of adequate calibre. If indicated, the posterior ethmoid air cells may be opened by penetrating the ground lamina of the middle turbinate. Dissection through these air cells leads to the sphenoid sinus, where again disease can be removed under direct vision.

Radiographic findings after ethmoidectomy

Postoperatively, the ethmoid sinus is best visualized using CT with a wide-window setting, to allow adequate visualization of any remaining bony septa as well as the interface between soft tissue, bone and air. The bony leaflets separating the ethmoid air cells are usually absent posterior to the ethmoid infundibulum (Figures 10.10. and 10.11). The middle turbinate may have been partially or completely resected. This deficit may extend back to the sphenoid sinus if such extensive surgery was performed. The middle turbinate may have been resected to provide access to the more posterior air cells and sometimes may be the only certain indicator that the patient has had an intranasal ethmoidectomy, especially if inadequate clinical details have been provided by the surgeon (Figures 10.12–10.16). Ideally, a remnant of the vertical plate of the middle turbinate should remain as a landmark indicating the site of the cribriform plate should revision surgery be needed (Figures 10.17 and 10.18). In some instances, partially resected middle turbinates may cause synechia or collapse against the lateral nasal wall, producing obstruction to the ostiomeatal unit (Figure 10.19).

The ideal result is a single well-aerated cavity. In the first 6 weeks following surgery there will be some opacification of the aerated cavity as a consequence of residual blood clot and edema of the remaining soft tissue. At a later stage, persistent opacification may represent scarring. This is usually of the same density as muscle and fails to enhance, unlike inflamed mucosa. Scar tissue can appear as thin strands of tissue filling the sinus lumen, as a solid mass or with a more nodular appearance.

The lamina papyracea should remain intact, although it may have been breached during the surgical procedure (Figure 10.20). This may lead to prolapse of the orbital fat into the ethmoid cavity, which may be tempting to avulse at revision surgery if not recognized as fat on CT (Figure 10.21). After some time, the medial wall of the orbit may collapse medially, reducing the lumen of the surgical defect and reversing the usual convexity of the intact lamina papyracea. The postoperative appearance may be mimicked by an orbital blow-out fracture or by hypertrophy of the extraocular muscles associated with hyperthyroidism. In the latter situation, the patient may have undergone orbital decompression; if so, the medial portion of the orbital floor will be absent.

Following surgery, the lamina papyracea, medial orbital wall, the roof of the ethmoid and any remaining bony septae will frequently be noted to be denser and sclerotic (Figures 10.12 and 10.22). This is usually secondary to reactive osteitis which on occasions may be extensive enough to obliterate the surgical defect.

The posterior ethmoid air cells are renowned for being a difficult and hazardous area for the surgeon to operate in, and it is possible for untouched air cells to contain residual disease despite the surgeon's report that all of the posterior air cells have been exenterated (Figure 10.18). Overzealous surgery in this area may lead to injury to surrounding vital anatomic structures, such as the optic nerve, the eyeball or even the internal carotid artery.

Following a transantral ethmoidectomy the postoperative radiologic features will include deficits of both the anterior and medial antral walls as well as the loss of a variable number of fine, bony leaflets separating the ethmoid air cells. The lamina papyracea should be intact unless the indication for surgery was to perform orbital decompression (Figure 10.9).

Following external ethmoidectomy a portion of the lamina papyracea will be noted to be absent on the CTs. The surgical defect is usually sharply demarcated, thereby differentiating it from the more gradual reduction of bone thickness resulting from an erosive process.

Following a transorbital ethmoidectomy for orbital decompression, the lamina papyracea should be deficient below the frontoethmoid suture line, as should the medial half of the orbital floor. The orbital fat should prolapse into the defect.

Following endoscopic sinus surgery the bony defects are usually confined to those sinus pre-chambers that were noted to be obstructed during the initial investigations. The entire ethmoid sinus area is replaced by a single large space after removal of the intervening septa. This often involves resection of the uncinate process, the ethmoid bulla and the creation of a wide middle meatal antrostomy. Some patients may have undergone more radical surgery previously and bony defects related to these procedures will remain evident (Figures 10.9–10.11 and 10.23).

FRONTAL SINUS TREPHINATION

Indication

Acute frontal sinusitis.

Technique

A short incision (1 cm) is made below the medial end of the eyebrow. The floor of the frontal sinus is perforated either with a drill or a hammer and gouge. The opening is enlarged sufficiently to allow drainage of the purulent secretions and to allow the insertion of an indwelling catheter for frequent irrigation of the sinus. The latter remains in place until the fluid used for irrigation passes through the frontal recess into the nose.

Radiographic findings

The radiographic features should reflect a resolving sinusitis with a small bony defect in the medial part of the floor of the frontal sinus (Figure 10.24).

EXTERNAL FRONTOETHMOIDECTOMY

Indications

Chronic frontoethmoid sinusitis, recurrent nasal polyposis, frontoethmoid mucoceles, complicated acute sinusitis. To provide access for transethmoidal hypophysectomy, dacrocystorhinostomy, and orbital decompression.

Technique

This procedure was described by both Lynch and Howarth. A temporary tarsorrhaphy is performed to protect the cornea. An incision is placed curving from below the medial margin of the eyebrow to pass midway between the medial canthus and the bridge of the nose. The procedure is similar to that of an external ethmoidectomy, except that it is extended to include resection of the floor of the frontal sinus and the middle turbinate. A silastic tube is often placed in the widened frontonasal duct to prevent stenosis and will remain in place for up to 3 months.

Radiographic findings

The radiographic features are similar to those of the external ethmoidectomy with the additional widening of the frontal recess and excision of the floor of the frontal sinus.

OSTEOPLASTIC FLAP WITH OBLITERATION OF FRONTAL SINUS

Indications

Chronic frontal sinusitis, excision of osteomata, excision of mucocele and repair of trauma.

Technique

A template of the frontal sinus is cut from a plain radiograph. A bicoronal flap is then elevated and the outline of the frontal sinus is marked onto the frontal bone. The bone of the anterior wall of the frontal sinus is then divided obliquely with a fissure burr and the intersinus septum divided with a chisel. The bony flap is then hinged forward on an intact inferiorly based pedicle of periosteum. Meticulous excision of all diseased tissue is essential and the sinus is obliterated with a free fat graft harvested from the anterior abdominal wall. The osteoplastic flap is then replaced.

Radiographic findings

Images of the frontal sinus following surgery will appear opaque. The outline of the sinus is often visible where the bone has been divided (Figure 10.25). In these patients, it can often be extremely difficult, because of the opacity, to distinguish changes that may occur as a consequence of recurrent disease. There are a variety of different but normal CT appearances that represent different stages of fibrosis of the obliterating fat graft. The bone flap should be examined with wide-window settings. This will also demonstrate the air-free frontal sinus. The sinus may appear to be air filled if it is only examined with narrow window settings. Ideally, the bone flap should have smooth edges and be aligned with the surrounding bone. With narrow-window examinations the fat should demonstrate a streaky appearance. This represents fibrosis in the graft. Complications include osteomyelitis of the bone flap, infection of the fat graft and mucocele formation. If the patient presents with recurrent symptoms, care must be taken to exclude inflammatory disease in the other paranasal sinuses. If a bony complication has developed, CT is of greater value than MR in demonstrating the lesion. The bone flap may be seen to be elevated or rotated, and there may be bone erosion or sequestrum formation. If the fat graft becomes infected it appears of a similar density to soft tissue rather than fat. This may become localized. If intracranial or intraorbital complications occur, they may be better visualized by MR.

LATERAL RHINOTOMY

Indications

Excision of inverted papilloma and other localized tumors such as malignant melanoma.

Technique

This procedure was first described in 1902 by Moure. The incision extends from the midpoint between the medial canthus and the bridge of the nose, along the natural skin crease of the nasojugal fold, around the alae of the nostrils and into the philtrum. The bony wall is exposed from the infraorbital canal to the frontoethmoid suture line. The lateral wall of the nose is excised *en bloc* by incisions (i) along the floor of the nose, opening the maxillary antrum; (ii) the anterior wall of the maxillary antrum is divided below the inferomedial angle; (iii) the nasal bone is divided up to the level of the frontonasal suture line, demarcating the level of the cribriform plate; (iv) the ethmoid arteries are ligated and the frontoethmoid suture line is divided to the posterior ethmoid artery, (the limit of safety to avoid damage to the optic nerve); (v) the orbital rim is divided with the lamina papyracea and the lateral wall removed in one piece. The amount of maxilla resected can be tailored depending on the pathology and the extent of the disease.

Radiographic findings

The radiographic deficit includes the absence of the medial wall of the orbit extending from the infraorbital canal to the frontoethmoidal suture line. A large nasoantral cavity is formed after the removal of the entire lateral wall of the nose including the middle and inferior turbinates (Figure 10.6).

MAXILLECTOMY

Indication

Malignancy involving the maxillary antrum.

Techniques

The incision used is similar to that used for the lateral rhinotomy, but it is extended along the margin of the lower lid, if the globe is being preserved, or along the margin of both eyelids, if the orbit is to be exenterated. The hard palate is divided in the midline, the orbital floor is then dissected free depending on the extent of the disease, the zygoma is divided, the lateral wall of the nose is divided below the frontoethmoid suture line, and finally the pterygoid plates are separated from the posterior aspect of the maxilla.

Radiographic findings

The postoperative appearance will depend on the extent of the surgery, that is either a partial or total maxillectomy. If the maxilla is removed in its entirety the pterygoid plates usually remain and may be identified on the images. Usually there is a clearly defined cavity which is sharply demarcated. Recurrent disease is indicated by the development of a soft-tissue mass or further bony erosion.

RADIOLOGIC APPEARANCES OF COMPLICATIONS FOLLOWING OF SURGERY

A knowledge of the neighboring structures of the paranasal sinuses, already described in detail, makes it understandable that there will be a certain morbidity from surgical injury to these structures. The task of the surgeon is further complicated by misleading variations in the anatomy and pneumatization or by anatomic landmarks that may be disguised by disease. Serious complications are rare but may occur even at the hands of the most experienced and well-trained surgeons. The prompt recognition of a complication and its appropriate management should allow the optimum conditions for recovery.

The complications of sinus surgery can be classified into minor and major complications. The minor complication include postoperative bleeding, hematoma, orbital emphysema, and scarring with obstruction of the ventilation and drainage pathways. The major complications include ocular or optic nerve injury, cerebrospinal fluid rhinorrhea, injury to the lacrimal apparatus, internal carotid artery injury and anosmia. Rare complications are brain injury, intracranial infection, brain abscess and meningitis.

Complications most commonly occur following intranasal polypectomy, intranasal ethmoidectomy and sphenoidectomy. The risks are greater if there has been prior surgery and some of the usual landmarks may have been removed. The complications will be discussed in relation to the nasal cavity, the orbit and optic nerve, the anterior cranial fossa and the sphenoid sinus relations – the internal carotid artery and the cavernous sinus.

Nasal cavity complications

A common and expected problem following intranasal procedures is haemorrhage. This is usually controlled with an intranasal pack which may be left in place for up to 48 hours. Plain gauze packs have a characteristic appearance if left in place during a postoperative scan, as can be seen in Figure 10.26. Some surgeons prefer to use ribbon gauze that has been impregnated with bismuth iodoform paraffin paste (BIPP). The heavy metal, bismuth, will cause widespread artifact if left in place during a postoperative scan. Even following its removal, small deposits of the bismuth paste will remain as small dense areas (Figure 10.27). Other later local complications include synechiae (adhesions) (Figure 10.28), collapse of the lateral wall of the nose (Figure 10.29) and lateralization of the middle turbinate causing obstruction of the frontal recess (Figure 10.19). The late complications include mucocele formation as a result of compartmentalization and obstruction to drainage (Figure 10.30).

Orbital complications include blindness and diplopia following injury to the optic nerve, the extraocular muscles or the orbital fat. The commonest cause of blindness is a retrobulbar hematoma, causing exophthalmos and stretching of the optic nerve. Rapid decompression of the hematoma may preserve optic function. Bilateral blindness has been reported following bilateral retrobulbar hematoma and also following bilateral optic nerve section. The optic nerve is particularly at risk if there is a large Onodi's cell extending laterally around the nerve (Figure 10.31). Hematoma will become evident on CT following the administration of intravenous contrast. Optic nerve section becomes apparent on visualizing the injured segment of the nerve.

The lamina papyracea may be injured during intranasal ethmoidectomy. This may occur when the uncinate process is resected to facilitate middle meatal antrostomy. Portions of the lamina papyracea may be inadvertently avulsed with nasal polyps allowing the orbital fat to prolapse into the nasal cavity (Figures 10.30 and 10.32). Subperiosteal hematoma may occur in the operative area. This becomes evident with periorbital ecchymosis and exophthalmos. CTs will demonstrate an enhancing lesion running alongside the medial orbital wall (Figure 10.20). The orbit may also be accidentally injured during a transantral ethmoidectomy. The orbital floor may be breached if mistaken for the ethmomaxillary plate (Figures 10.33–10.35).

Anterior cranial fossa injury

To avoid injury to the anterior cranial fossa, particular care is needed in dissecting medial to the vertical plate of the middle turbinate. This bony attachment is on the border of the cribriform plate, and careless dissection or avulsion of the middle turbinate may lead to a cerebrospinal fluid leak and the risk of meningitis (Figure 10.36). If such an accident occurs and is recognized intraoperatively then the defect should be repaired immediately. If the defect is recognized later, the intervention of a neurosurgeon may be required. The ethmoid fovea which roofs the ethmoid air cells, is thicker then the cribriform plate but it is still vulnerable to injury. Care must be taken in operating anywhere near the roof of the anterior ethmoid (the floor of the anterior cranial fossa), and rocking of the perpendicular plate of the ethmoid during its removal in a septoplasty should also be avoided. The site of bony defects becomes evident on coronal CTs, allowing accurate targetting of repair, should this be necessary.

Sphenoid sinus, cavernous sinus and carotid artery injury

Careful assessment of the anatomy of the sphenoid sinus and its vascular relations should help to prevent massive intraoperative hemorrhage. CT has a greater role in the prevention of such catastrophes than in their immediate diagnosis and management. The position of the internal carotid artery can be identified and any bony dehiscences will be noted prior to commencing surgery. When the surgeon plans to enter the sphenoid sinus, both coronal and axial CTs should be obtained. Axial CTs are superior for showing the relationship of the optic nerve to the posterior ethmoid and sphenoid sinuses, as well as the relationship of the carotid artery to the sphenoid sinus.

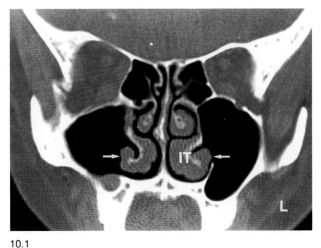

10.1

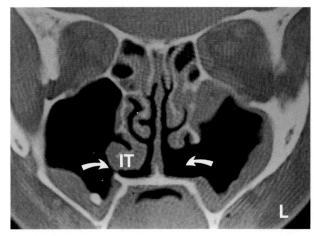

10.2

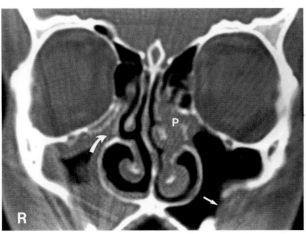

10.3

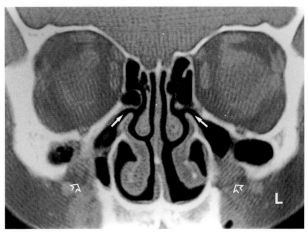

10.4

Figure **10.1**

Intranasal antrostomy. This coronal CT scan demonstrates bilateral intranasal antrostomies with large hypertrophied inferior turbinates (IT), occluding the antrostomy sites (arrows). Note on the right side how the medial antral wall has been resected to the level of the floor of the nasal cavity, whereas on the left a considerable amount of the medial wall remains.

Figure **10.3**

Residual disease following Caldwell–Luc procedures. This patient presented with persistent left malar pain and nasal obstruction despite bilateral Caldwell–Luc procedures. This coronal CT scan demonstrates a large polyp in the left middle meatus (P) blocking the ostiomeatal complex. Excision of the polyp and reopening of the natural ostium of the maxillary sinus led to resolution of the patient's symptoms. Note the dehiscent bone in the area of the sublabial antrostomy on the left (arrow). The mucosal thickening in the right maxillary sinus is consistent with chronic sinusitis. Note the blocked infundibulum on this side (curved arrow).

Figure **10.2**

Bilateral intranasal antrostomies. This coronal CT scan demonstrates wide bilateral intranasal antrostomies (curved arrows). The antrostomy on the left is widely patent, whereas the antrostomy on the right is totally blocked by a grossly enlarged inferior turbinate (IT). There is mucosal disease in both maxillary sinuses. Failure of this procedure is due to the inflammatory disease obstruction the ostiomeatal complex.

Figure **10.4**

Bilateral Caldwell–Luc procedures (open arrows): CT scan. Although this patient has patent ostiomeatal complex bilaterally (arrows), scarring and compartmentalization have resulted in persistent symptoms of pain and sinus infection.

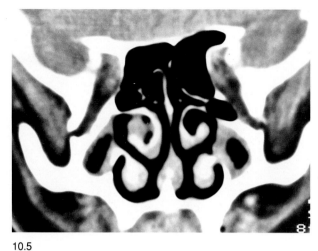

10.5

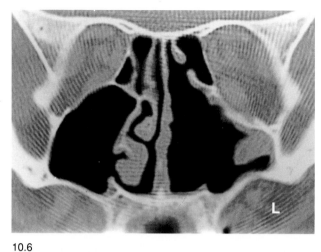

10.6

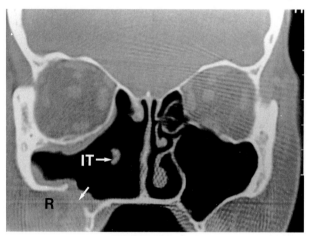

10.7

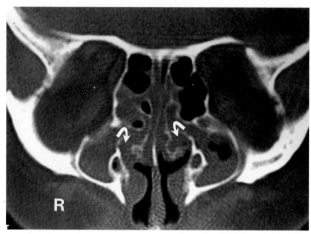

10.8

Figure 10.5

Postoperative hypoplasia of the maxillary sinus: CT scan. There is thickening of the bony walls and the mucous membranes at the expense of the sinus lumen.

Figure 10.6

Intranasal ethmoidectomy with exenteration of the lateral nasal wall. This coronal CT scan demonstrates the defect following resection of the lateral nasal wall and intranasal ethmoidectomy. The resulting surgical defect allows the entire maxillary sinus to open into the empty and capacious nasal cavity.

Figure 10.7

Transantral ethmoidectomy. This coronal CT scan demonstrates a clean ethmoid cavity following a right transantral ethmoidectomy. There is minimal residual mucosal thickening within the maxillary sinus which is probably of no clinical significance. The defect in the anterior wall (arrow) represents the sublabial antrostomy. The middle turbinate has been removed. A remnant of the inferior turbinate (IT) appears to be 'floating' in an otherwise large and empty, aerated cavity.

Figure 10.8

Functional endoscopic ethmoidectomy. Preoperative scan. This coronal CT scan demonstrates bilateral pansinusitis. Both ostiomeatal complexes are blocked (curved arrows), and secondary infection has occurred in the maxillary sinuses.

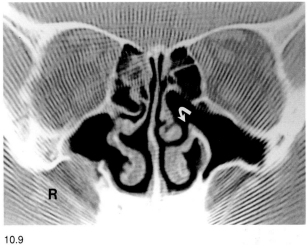

10.9

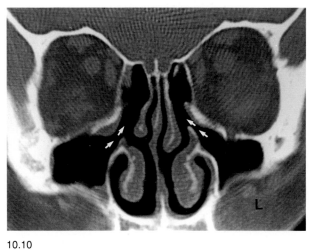

10.10

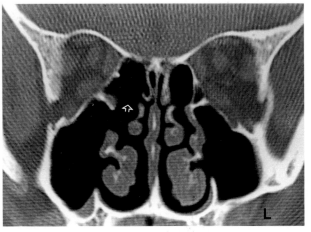

10.11

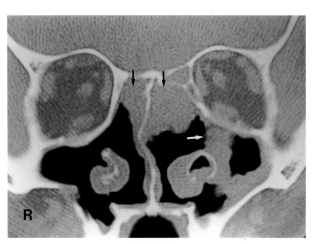

10.12

Figure **10.9**

Functional endoscopic ethmoidectomy. Postoperative scan of the same patient as in Figure 10.8. This coronal CT scan shows the surgical defect following a left functional endoscopic ethmoidectomy. The uncinate process has been resected and the natural ostium of the maxillary sinus enlarged (curved arrow). Note how the secondary infection within the maxillary sinus has resolved following the restoration of ventilation and drainage.

Figure **10.10**

Postoperative scans following intranasal ethmoidectomy. This coronal CT scan taken following functional endoscopic sinus surgery shows that a complete bilateral anterior ethmoidectomy has been performed. The ostiomeatal complexes are patent (arrows). The uncinate process has been completely removed on the right and partially resected on the left.

Figure **10.11**

Postoperative scan following intranasal ethmoidectomy. In this CT scan which is more posterior than Figure 10.10, the right basal lamella has been perforated (open arrow), ventilating the posterior ethmoid air cells with good result. There is no evidence of recurrent disease. Note the bilateral intranasal antrostomies.

Figure **10.12**

Complete intranasal ethmoidectomy with residual disease: CT scan. This patient, with recurrent nasal polyps, has had bilateral intranasal ethmoidectomies, bilateral intranasal antrostomies, a right Caldwell–Luc procedure and resection of both middle turbinates. There is recurrent inflammatory disease in the anterior ethmoid along the roof of the nasal cavity (black arrows). Note the inflammatory tissue blocking the natural ostium of the left maxillary sinus (white arrow) and the mucosal disease within the sinus proper.

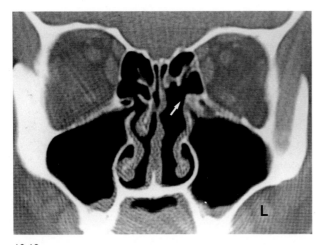

10.13

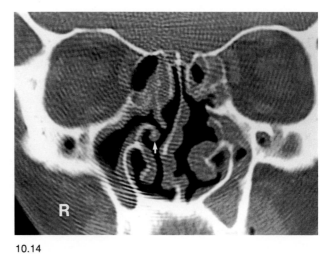

10.14

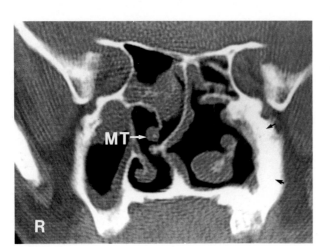

10.15

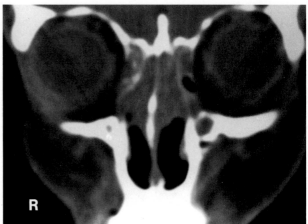

10.16

Figure **10.13**

Resection of the middle turbinate: CT scan. This patient has had an incomplete left intranasal ethmoidectomy (arrow), with resection of the vertical plate of the middle turbinate. Note the blocked left ostiomeatal complex.

Figure **10.14**

Bilateral incomplete ethmoidectomy with residual disease. This coronal CT scan demonstrates that the left middle turbinate has been resected, and the right middle turbinate has been partially resected. An incomplete ethmoidectomy has been performed. Note the inverted uncinate process (arrow). Also note the fibrous and osseous proliferation in the left maxillary sinus.

Figure **10.15**

Bilateral incomplete ethmoidectomy with residual disease. This coronal CT scan, taken posterior to Figure 10.14, demonstrates that the middle turbinate on the left has been resected. Note the bilateral posterior ethmoid disease and the intact posterior portion of the middle turbinate (MT) on the right. There is marked sclerosis of the lateral wall of the left maxillary sinus (arrows).

Figure **10.16**

Recurrent nasal polyps. This patient with the ASA triad had undergone multiple intranasal polypectomies. The soft-tissue mass filling the upper half of each nasal cavity represents recurrent polyps. In these patients, the CT scan is primarily of use to the surgeon in identifying any remaining bony structures, and in demonstrating any potential danger areas such as dehiscences of the orbital wall.

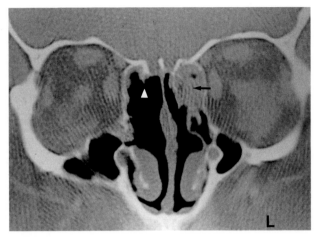

10.17

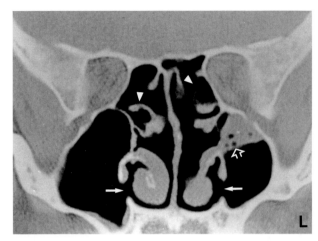

10.18

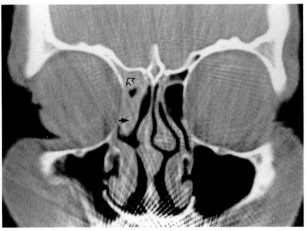

10.19

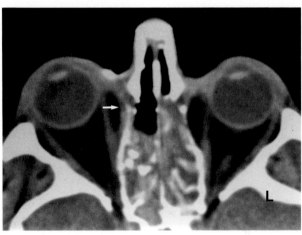

10.20

Figure **10.17**

Incomplete ethmoidectomy with recurrent polyps: CT scan. This patient has undergone a complete right intranasal ethmoidectomy with excision of the right middle turbinate (arrowhead). The left ethmoidectomy is incomplete and there is residual polypoid disease in the anterior ethmoid (black arrow).

Figure **10.18**

Bilateral incomplete ethmoidectomy with recurrent polyps. This is a more posterior CT scan of the patient shown in Figure 10.17. The posterior ethmoidectomies are incomplete (arrowheads). Bilateral patent intranasal antrostomies are present (arrows). The air bubbles within the 'soft-tissue' mass in the roof of the left maxillary sinus identifies this mass as thick mucus (open arrow).

Figure **10.19**

Lateralized middle turbinate. This coronal CT scan demonstrates lateralization of the right middle turbinate (arrow) which occurred following surgery. Fracture of the vertical insertion of the middle turbinate has resulted in its collapse with obstruction and disease of the frontal recess (open arrow).

Figure **10.20**

Breach of the lamina papyracea and subperiosteal intraorbital hemorrhage. This axial CT scan demonstrates a small subperiosteal hematoma that followed breach of the lamina papyracea during intranasal ethmoidectomy (arrow). The radio-opaque material in the nasal cavity is the remains of bismuth iodoform paraffin paste from an intranasal pack that was placed postoperatively.

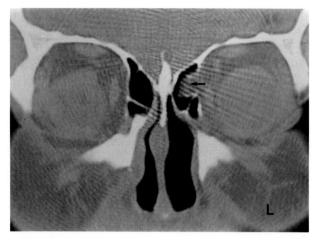

10.21

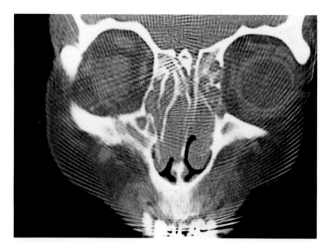

10.22

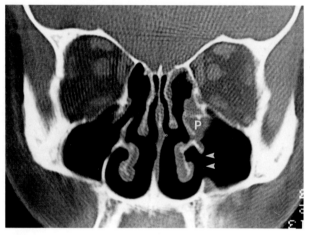

10.23

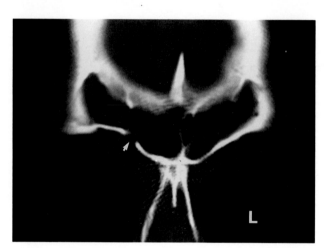

10.24

Figure **10.21**

Defect of the lamina papyracea. This coronal CT scan demonstrates orbital fat prolapsing through a defect in the left lamina papyracea (arrow), following ethmoidectomy.

Figure **10.22**

Residual anterior ethmoid disease. This CT scan demonstrates the defects in the lamina papyracea on the left side. Note the recurrent polyps in the ethmoid cavity and sclerosis of the lamina papyracea on the right side.

Figure **10.23**

A large polyp (P) is seen in the ethmoid infundibulum. This patient continued to be symptomatic despite previous sinus surgery (arrowheads).

Figure **10.24**

Frontal sinus trephine. This anterior coronal CT scan demonstrates a defect in the floor of the right frontal sinus following a recent trephine (arrow). Both frontal sinuses are opacified as the result of pansinusitis.

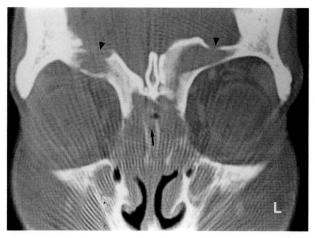

10.25

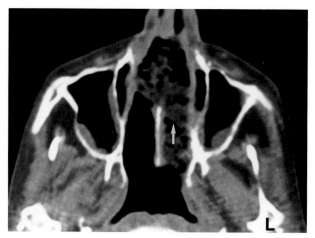

10.26

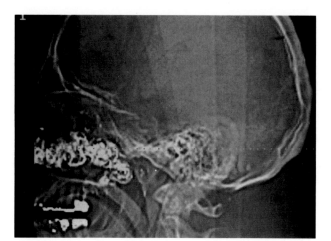

10.27

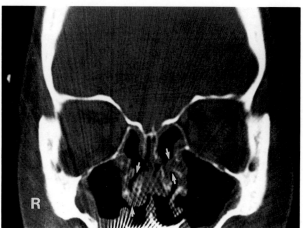

10.28

Figure 10.25

Osteoplastic flap. This coronal CT scan demonstrates the surgical defect of the osteoplastic flap used for the excision of a frontal sinus mucocele. There are large surgical defects in the roof of the frontal sinus (arrowheads). A small silastic tube is seen displaced medially between the frontal recess and the nasal septum (arrow).

Figure 10.26

Gauze nasal pack. This CT scan demonstrates an area filled irregularly with air and soft tissue (arrow). This is a gauze pack used to control epistaxis. It should not be mistaken for inflammatory disease. This patient has had a radical ethmoidectomy in the past.

Figure 10.27

Bismuth iodoform paraffin paste pack. This lateral CT view of the skull shows radio-opaque mass of a bismuth iodoform paraffin paste, intranasal pack which is placed *in situ* postoperatively to control hemorrhage.

Figure 10.28

Synechia. This coronal CT scan demonstrates that this patient has had both intranasal antrostomies and intranasal ethmoidectomies in the past. Synechia can be seen bridging between the lateral nasal wall and the middle turbinates (arrows).

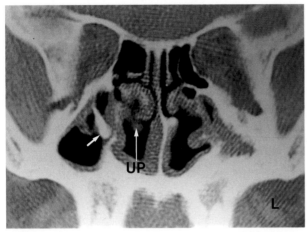

10.29

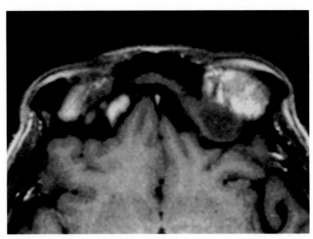

10.30

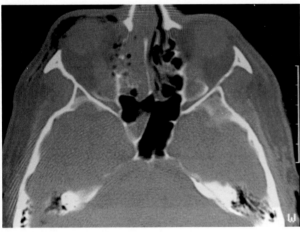

10.31

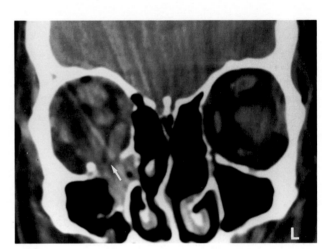

10.32

Figure **10.29**

Fracture of the lateral nasal wall. This coronal CT scan demonstrates that the inferior turbinates have been resected too close to the lateral nasal wall (arrow). The lateral nasal wall has fractured and been displaced laterally, causing occlusion of the ostiomeatal complex and associated scarring and deformity of the partially resected inferior turbinate and uncinate process (UP).

Figure **10.30**

Frontal sinus mucocele. This axial T1-weighted MR scan demonstrates a hypointense mass in the left orbit. This was a frontal sinus mucocele which developed as the result of an unsuccessful obliterative procedure on the left frontal sinus.

Figure **10.31**

Orbital emphysema. Immediately following endoscopic sinus surgery, the patient developed proptosis. The axial CT scans demonstrate air in the orbit.

Figure **10.32**

Intraoperative orbital injury. This coronal CT scan shows the site at which the surgeon fractured through the floor of the orbit (arrow). The higher density of the right orbital contents results from intraorbital bleeding. Note the small bubble of air seen in the superior aspect of the orbit.

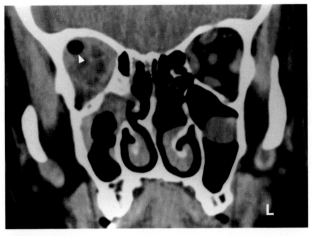

10.33

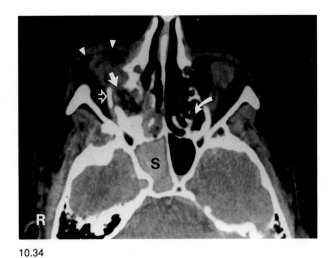

10.34

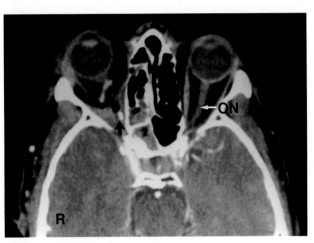

10.35

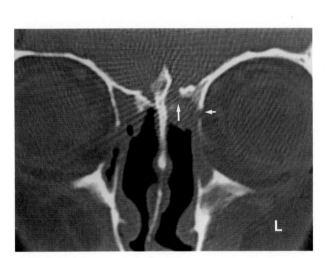

10.36

Figure **10.33**

Intraoperative orbital injury. This coronal CT scan (more posterior than Figure 10.32), demonstrates the orbital emphysema more clearly in the superior aspect of the orbit (arrowhead). The effects of hemorrhage, causing higher density of the right orbital contents, are more marked.

Figure **10.34**

Intraoperative orbital injury. This axial CT scan of the same patient as in Figures 10.32 and 10.33 also demonstrates orbital emphysema (arrowheads). The optic nerve has been transected (white arrow) by a large displaced portion of the lateral wall of the superior recess of the maxillary sinus (open arrow) through which the orbit was entered. The normal left superior recess of the maxillary sinus is shown (curved arrow). Note the hemorrhage in the sphenoid sinus (S).

Figure **10.35**

Intraoperative orbital injury. This axial CT scan of the same patient as in Figure 10.32, clearly shows the difference between the intact optic nerve on the left (ON), and the transected nerve on the right. There is retro-orbital hemorrhage adjacent to a displaced bone fragment (arrow).

Figure **10.36**

Fracture of the cribriform plate. This coronal CT scan was obtained following bilateral complete intranasal ethmoidectomies. The cribriform plate has been avulsed at the insertion of the left middle turbinate which was removed during the procedure (arrow). There is also a small defect in the left lamina papyracea (arrowhead).

11

Basic principles of Magnetic Resonance Imaging of the paranasal sinuses

Magnetic Resonance (MR) imaging is a complex process that involves magnets, radiofrequency coils and a computer information processing system similar to that used in computed tomography (CT). This chapter provides a simplified introduction to the basic physics and the technological aspects of MR.

MAGNETS

Three types of magnets are used for MR: the main magnet, the gradient coil and the shim coils.

The main magnet consists of a superconducting magnet, a resistive magnet or a permanent magnet. A permanent magnet is large, and the initial installation is expensive; however, the maintenance costs of this type of magnet are low. In resistive or super-conductive magnets the magnetic field is maintained by electric power or cryogens. These magnets are made from a solenoidal material and the patient lies along the direction of the magnetic field. Super-conductive electromagnets are cooled with both liquid helium and liquid nitrogen. This makes maintenance expensive. However, with their high field strengths and field homogeneity, superconductive magnets, are the best suited for clinical imaging.

The gradient coil varies the magnetic field through x-, y- and z-axes in a systematic fashion so that scans are possible in any plane and the signals received can be spatially localized.

The shim coils are resistive electromagnetic coils that make the magnetic field uniform by removing any inhomogeneities in the magnetic field.

RADIOFREQUENCY (RF) COILS

Radiofrequency coils transmit radiofrequency pulses through the patient to excite the nuclei. The larger coils transmit the pulses through the patient and the smaller surface coils receive the MR signals that are created following stimulation of the nuclei. These coils vary in size depending upon the part of the body being examined. Using an appropriately sized coil for the part being examined is important, and close proximity to the small field of view chosen prevents loss of the signals emitted from the excited nuclei.

The human body is ideally suited for MR because it has an abundant supply of hydrogen in the form of water or fat. When these hydrogen nuclei are placed in a strong magnetic field, they undergo a 'spin' or excitation. Not all nuclei 'spin' when placed in a magnetic field. Those nuclei that have an odd number of protons or an odd number of neutrons possess an angular momentum and so will spin. Among the naturally occurring elements that have an odd number of protons or neutrons are hydrogen (one proton and no neutrons), sodium-23, carbon-13 and phosphorus-31. Hydrogen atoms are the most abundant element in the human body, and thus serve as the ideal ingredient for interaction with the applied external magnetic field. Rotational motion of the atom is essential; without it, a nucleus will not be able to precess (spin) when placed in an external magnetic field.

When there is no external magnetic field, the unpaired protons are randomly oriented and the net magnetization is zero (Figure 11.1). When the nuclei are placed in a strong static external magnetic field, slightly more than 50% of them align in the direction of the applied external magnetic field, i.e. parallel (lower energy), and fewer protons assume the antiparallel (higher energy) direction. There is constant interaction between the protons in the higher energy, the protons in the lower energy, and the adjacent macromolecules. This results in 'equilibrium' — a net magnetization that is parallel to the external magnetic field. The protons continue to spin around the axis of the external magnetic field. This rate of precession is proportional to the external magnetic field. The net magnetization, i.e. longitudinal magnetization, in the tissues cannot be measured until it is tipped into transverse direction. 'Equilibrium' in the tissue is disturbed by the application of a radiofrequency pulse of a certain amplitude and strength, i.e. the Larmor frequency, the frequency at which magnetic reasonance in a nucleus can be excited and detected. The Larmor Frequency determines the frequency to which the receiver coils should be tuned to receive the MR signal from the patient.

MR image production and contrast are dependent on several factors. Some of these factors characterize the tissue being examined (T1, T2 and proton density, which is the density of the proton spins) and contribute to tissue contrast. These parameters are unique to the tissue being examined and can only be altered by the use of paramagnetic agents. Most of these paramagnetic agents exert their effects by reducing the proton relaxation time or by altering the proton density. The other parameters that can be altered to affect signal intensity include repetition time (TR), echo time (TE), flip angle, field of view, matrix size and slice thickness. Some of these parameters will be discussed later in this chapter to better explain MR.

In summary, three types of electromagnetic fields are necessary for MR:

i   a static magnetic field to align the protons;
ii   a gradient magnetic field, which determines the spatial location of the signals received;
iii   a radiofrequency pulse to disturb the magnetic momentum of the protons.

RADIOFREQUENCY PULSE AND FLIP ANGLE

A radiofrequency (RF) pulse that flips or tips the longitundinal magnetization into transverse magnetization is a 90° RF pulse. The angle through which the longitudinal magnetization rotates to change its direction is called the flip angle (Figure 11.2). For example, an RF pulse that converts a longitudinal magnetization to a transverse magnetization has a flip angle of 90°, whilst an RF pulse that inverts longitudinal magnetization is a 180° RF pulse. The protons precess in the direction of the magnetic field at Larmor frequency after flipping into the transverse direction. The magnetic field continues to change with the precession of the nuclei. This induces in the

reciever coil an electrical voltage proportional to the strength of the transverse magnetization, constituting an MR signal. The MR signal is made of variable signal intensities, and an MR image is formed by these complex signals.

T1 RELAXATION TIME

The longitudinal magnetization recovery, i.e. the T1 relaxation time, is due to the transfer of energy to the surrounding tissues from the precessing nuclei. This is also referred to as 'spin-lattice relaxation'. Following excitation by a 90° RF pulse, the precessing or the excited nucleus tries to gain 'equilibrium', to realign with the static magnetic field. In liquids, hydrogen protons move very easily so there are fewer protons that fall in and out of the Larmor frequency. The longitudinal magnetization recovery is also slow for liquids, so the T1 relaxation time is long for liquids and they are dark on T1-weighted images. In solids, more protons precess at Larmor frequency, because the protons are not free to move easily. A tissue with a short T1 relaxation time, such as fat, rapidly recovers longitudinal magnetization and is bright on T1-weighted images (Figures 11.3 and 11.4). The T1 relaxation time is short for fat, hemorrhage, proteinaceous cysts and gadolinium-infused tissues. Liquids, edema and tumors have long T1 relaxation times. The gray and white matter of brain have intermediate signal intensity.

T2 RELAXATION TIME

When the 90° RF pulse is turned off, the protons that are precessing in the transverse plane slowly lose their momentum and start to dephase because there are some changes in the local magnetic field. These dephasing protons eventually realign with the external magnetic field. The decrease in the transverse magnetization is exponential and is called the free induction decay (FID). The rate of this decay of transverse to longitudinal magnetization states is called the T2 relaxation time (Figure 11.5). Some protons precess quickly, while others precess at a slow rate. The T2 relaxation time represents the decay due to the difference between protons in the precessional frequency, which results in loss of phase coherence. It is related to the static magnetic field and the magnetic field that each proton creates and is called the 'spin–spin relaxation'. Structures with long T2 relaxation time are fluid, edema and tumor, and these appear as bright signals. Tendons, muscles and cartilages have a short T2 relaxation time, appear dark and are of low signal intensity.

PULSE SEQUENCES

The pulse sequences are governed by the radio-frequency pulse used, the gradient manipulation done to select slices and the spatial resolution. Some of the sequences used for clinical imaging are spin-echo, inversion-recovery and gradient sequences. These sequences are appropriate for clinical imaging because minimal time is lost between stimulation of the tissue and the image production. Moreover, in addition to yielding an image that is diagnostically acceptable, these imaging sequences are performed with the least amount of discomfort to the patient.

SPIN-ECHO SEQUENCES

This is the most common pulse sequence used in clinical imaging. Initially, a 90° RF pulse is transmitted to flip the protons spinning in the longitudinal plane into the transverse plane. This is followed by a 180° RF pulse (phase reversal) which is necessary for rephasing the transverse magnetization. The signal is measured during the rephasing of the transverse magnetization. This is followed by a second 90° RF pulse and the sequence is repeated. The time interval between two consecutive 90° RF pulses is the repetition time (TR) (Figure 11.6). If a spin-echo sequence has a short TR (400–600 ms) between two consecutive 90° RF pulses and the echo time (TE) is kept short (<20 ms) so that only T1 signals are obtained, then the sequence is called *T1-weighted*. The echo time (TE) is the interval between the peak of the 90° RF pulse and the detection of the MR signal (Figure 11.6). If the TE is lengthened, then the protons will have time to dephase and the T2 relaxation effects will be seen.

T1-weighted images are obtained using short TR and short TE settings. This makes it possible to differentiate two tissues which have different signal intensities at short TR times but have almost similar intensity at long TR times. Hence TR controls T1-weighting (Figure 11.3 and 11.4).

A proton-density sequence is when all the T1 recovery is complete and T2 decay is minimal. These are called spin-density weighted images, and they require a long TR and a short TE. The proton density is dependent on the amount of water, that is the number of available hydrogen protons. The greater the proton density, the stronger will be the MR signal. The greater the difference in the proton density of adjacent tissues, the better the tissue contrast. Cysts, water and edema are hyperintense (bright) on proton-density sequences, and bone, air, cartilage and tendons are hypointense (dark) on these sequences. Bone and air are seen as signal void areas or black on MR images.

T2-weighted sequences are obtained using a long TR (1500–3000 ms) and a long TE (60–100 ms). Tissues with a long T2 relaxation time are better differentiated on T2-weighted sequences. The longer the TE, the greater the T2 effects of a tissue will be noted. Tissues with a long T2 relaxation time are hyperintense (bright) on T2-weighted sequences, because less decay of the transverse magnetization would have occurred at a given time. Tissues with a short T2 are hypointense (dark) on T2-weighted sequence, as most of the T2 effect is lost before the signal is received (Figure 11.5). In most instances, T1-weighted sequences are best for the delineation of anatomic structures and T2-weighted sequences for the assessment of pathology.

INVERSION RECOVERY SEQUENCES

Inversion recovery (IR) sequences involve initial excitation of the nuclei by a 180° RF pulse. This inverts the longitudinal magnetization. After a pause (TI inversion time) when some recovery of longitudinal magnetization is occurring, a 90° pulse is applied to flip the longitudinal magnetization to transverse magnetization. After another small pause (TR), a second 180° pulse is applied, following which the MR signal is measured. The short-TI IR (STIR) sequences are used to nullify the effects of fat, as the bright signals of fat often gives rise to artifacts during MR imaging.

GRADIENT-ECHO SEQUENCE

In gradient-echo imaging the 180° pulses are replaced by gradient reversals. If the 90° pulse is also replaced by a flip angle that is less than 90° then most of the longitudinal magnetization is left undisturbed and one does not have to wait for T1 signals. The RF pulse of less than 90° can be applied (TR) after the signal is obtained. Thus, in gradient-echo sequences, the contrast and signals are manipulated by changing the TR, TE and the flip angles of the RF pulse. If a flip angle of greater than 45° is used with a short TE, the sequences appear more T1-weighted. With a flip angle of less than 20° the images are more T2-weighted in appearance. The advantages of using a gradient-echo sequence is its rapid acquisition of MR images. Differentiation between flowing blood and thrombosed vessels is possible as blood flow is seen as bright signals. Hemosiderin and other substances with strong paramagnetic properties appear dark on gradient-echo sequences. These sequences are more sensitive in identifying punctate calcifications due to the magnetic susceptibility differences between normal tissue and calcification. Among fast imaging sequences that are used for clinical imaging are gradient-recalled acquisition in steady state (GRASS) and fast-low-angled shot (FLASH).

IMAGE RECONSTRUCTION

The MR signal obtained is amplified and received by a computer. This information of several signal intensities is converted into an image by a complex mathematical analysis process. There are at least two basic methods that are used: two- or three-dimensional fast Fourier imaging method and the projection reconstruction method. The two-dimensional Fourier analysis is one of the popular methods for MR imaging. This technique is used to generate an image from the signal intensities acquired from a small volume of tissue.

Initially two-dimensional Fourier analysis requires 'selective excitation' of a layer of tissue, by applying a weak magnetic field gradient in one plane. This selection can be in any plane. For an image in the axial plane, the slice selection gradient is applied in the z-axis. If the gradient is applied in the x- or y-direction the scans will be in the sagittal or in the coronal plane, respectively (Figure 11.7). Thus MR imaging is possible in any plane without the patient having to assume an uncomfortable position. The thickness of the slice depends on the gradient chosen.

Once the layer that is to be excited is chosen, then the frequency and the phase encoding gradients in the remaining two planes (x-axis for frequency and y-axis for phase encoding to obtain an axial image) should be done. Frequency encoding involves the display of several frequencies arising from various sites in a volume of tissue, for example in the x-direction for axial scans. Phase encoding, in the y-axis for axial scans, represents the spatial resolution along the chosen axis and is directly proportional to the number of 90° pulses with different phase-encoding gradients. Multisection acquisitions using two-dimensional Fourier transformation is the ideal method, as the information from several sections is obtained, while the frequency is shifted to excite a different section (Figure 11.8).

MAGNETIC RESONANCE IMAGING VERSUS COMPUTED TOMOGRAPHY

Both these technical advances in imaging have made it possible to diagnose patients efficiently. As it stands, CT and MR are two cross-sectional imaging modalities that are complementary to one another. There are several advantages and disadvantages to both these modalities.

Magnetic Resonance

The imaging can be done in any plane without moving the patient, or making the patient assume any uncomfortable position. It does not involve ionizing radiation and to date there is no evidence of any deleterious effects from strong magnetic fields.

Cortical bone, small metal clips, etc. do not cause artifacts in MR imaging.

MR gives superior resolution of soft-tissue contrast than CT. As MR involves direct interaction between the applied magnetic field and the tissue, certain tissue characterization and metabolic changes from disease can be deduced from a combination of MR spectroscopy and imaging.

Drawbacks to Magnetic Resonance

There are however several drawbacks to imaging with MR. Some patients, such as those who are claustrophobic, are not able to tolerate the length of procedure, others cannot tolerate the noise caused by the gradient coils during scanning. As the scanning time is lengthy (approximately 45 minutes to an hour for a head scan), motion and respiration artifacts degrade the images.

Large ferromagnetic agents and prostheses do degrade images, and patients with pacemakers, aneurysm clips and cochlear transplants are a definite contraindication to MR scanning. Most medical accessories such as wheel-chairs and intravenous poles have to be modified if they are to accompany a patient near the scanner.

CT is sensitive to small calcifications and subtle bony lesions. In contrast, MR does not image cortical bone and calcifications, tumors that are characterized by calcifications such as chondrogenic tumors and other bone or calcifying lesions can be misinterpreted on MR images. A wide variety of pathologic tissue and normal structures can have identical T1 and T2 relaxation times, and both these properties in a tissue can alter. The length of T1 and T2 relaxation times are not reliable for differentiating benign from malignant lesions.

CONTRAST-ENHANCED IMAGING

One of the distinct advantages of MR over CT is its superior resolution of soft-tissue contrast, which made most investigators feel that intravenous contrast media would not be necessary. It is now recognized, however, that intravenous contrast improves tissue contrast and is useful in intracranial and in spinal pathology. Contrast agents significantly improve lesion detectability and also increase the possibility of seeing lesions that were not well delineated in the precontrast study. Unlike the contrast agents that are directly visualized in CT, the paramagnetic agents that are used in MR imaging are not visualized directly. Instead, the agents primarily affect the proton density and the proton relaxation times, thus improving the contrast between normal and diseased tissues.

Like most contrast media that are used for conventional radiography, the paramagnetic agents should have certain standard properties, including the following.

i They should be stable, non-toxic and excreted rapidly without any deleterious effects to the organ that excretes the media.

ii They should be able to produce the necessary effects in the tissues, making it possible to image within a short time.

iii They should alter the tissue relaxation rates at non-toxic dosages.

The magnetopharmaceuticals used in imaging exhibit their paramagnetic properties due to the unpaired electrons in the outer shell.

They remain in the extracellular compartments and have large magnetic moments; nuclei in close proximity to them exhibit a decrease in their T1 and T2 relaxation times. Agents that effectively reduce the T1 relaxation times are best visualized on T1-weighted sequences, and those that reduce the T2-relaxation on T2-weighted sequences. Not uncommonly, both T1 and T2 relaxation times are simultaneously affected.

The most common paramagnetic agent used in clinical imaging is gadolinium-diethylenetriamine-penta-acetic acid (Gd-DTPA). Gadolinium is a rare earth element, with seven unpaired electrons, which exhibits definite paramagnetic properties. Free gadolinium is toxic and not suitable for clinical use. However, chelating gadolinium with DTPA, the gadolinium retains its paramagnetic properties, is stable and is rendered metabolically inert.

Gd-DTPA dimeglumine is the form that is injected intravenously. The meglumine ion dissociates from the Gd-DTPA immediately. The Gd-DTPA remains in the extracellular compartment, not crossing the blood–brain barrier, and, like other paramagnetic agents, exerts its effects there. It is excreted by glomerular filtration in an unaltered state by the kidneys.

The usual routine includes T1 and T2-weighted scans prior to contrast administration, followed by a slow infusion of Gd-DTPA (dosage 0.2 ml/kg of body weight to a maximum of 20 ml). The T1-weighted sequences are repeated within the next 1.5 hours, as the effects of Gd-DTPA are best noted within the first hour.

Most adverse reactions occur immediately after injection. The common side effects include nausea, vomiting, headaches, dizziness and pain at injection site. Gd-DTPA is known to decrease the threshold for convulsions and should be used with caution in patients with a history of convulsive disorder. Hemolysis of red blood cells with transient increase in the serum iron and bilirubin levels have been noted. Theroretically speaking, Gd-DTPA can accelerate the hemolytic effects in patients with hemolytic anemia.

There are several structures that normally enhance following the administration of Gd-DTPA.

These include the pituitary gland and its stalk, the cavernous sinus, the choroid plexus and the grey matter, intracranially.

The extracranial structures that enhance are the nasal turbinates and the sinonasal mucosa. In paranasal sinus imaging tumors show only moderate enhancement compared with the intense enhancement exhibited by normal tissue. Scar tissue and sinonasal secretions do not enhance. One has to be careful in interpreting scans following enhancement with Gd-DTPA. As the tumor enhances, the fat–tumor interface may be obscured and there is a likelihood of misinterpreting the lesion to be larger than its actual size.

ROUTINE TECHNIQUE IN PARANASAL SINUS IMAGING

Preliminary T1-weighted MR scans are obtained in the axial plane. The slices are 5 mm thick and the interslice distance is 1 mm. The coronal scans are localized from the axial study. Proton density and the T2-weighted scans are obtained in the coronal plane, as this is the ideal plane for paranasal sinus imaging. The sagittal plane is excellent for assessing the midline structures, the cribriform plate, and the sphenoid sinus and its drainage pathway. T1-weighted sequences are ideal for anatomic details and are done in the axial and coronal planes if this is necessary.

For T1-weighted images, the TR is short and is 300–500 ms, and TE is 20–35 ms. T2-weighted sequences are obtained with a long TR (1800–200 ms) and a TE of 20–35 ms for the first echo (also called the proton-density weighted image) and 70–120 ms for the second echo. These parameters are dependent upon the size of the magnet.

Scans are tailored so that the imaging time is not excessively long.

Gadolinium-enhanced MR scans are obtained within 30 minutes of injection. T1-weighted sequences are obtained, to evaluate the shortening of the T1 relaxation time.

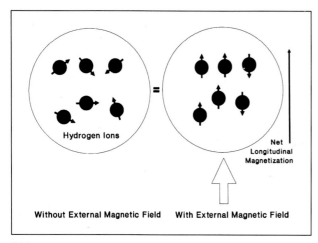

11.1

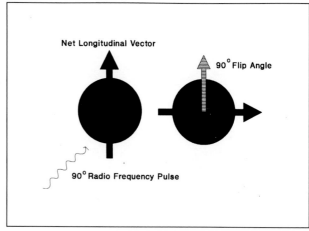

11.2

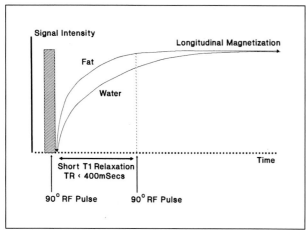

11.3

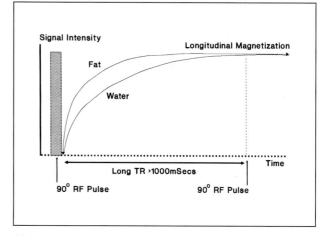

11.4

Figure **11.1**

Without an external magnetic field the orientation of the hydrogens ions is random. Following the application of a magnetic field, the hydrogen ions align with the direction of the applied magnetic field or against it. The net longitudinal magnetization is orientated in the same plane as the applied static magnetic field.

Figure **11.2**

A 90° radiofrequency pulse applied at the Larmor frequency will tip the net longitudinal vector into the transverse plane. The transverse magnetization is responsible for the MR signal. The angle through which the net longitudinal vector rotates to change direction is the flip angle.

Figure **11.3**

The repetition time (TR) for the 90° radiofrequency pulse is short. Fat has a short T1-relaxation time and recovers longitudinal magnetization rapidly. Hence fat is bright on T1-weighted images. In order to differentiate fat from water, which has a long T1 relaxation time, a short TR is needed (see Figure 11.4).

Figure **11.4**

When the TR from the 90° radiofrequency pulse is long, the difference in the T1 values of water and fat is small and these two structures will not be differentiated.

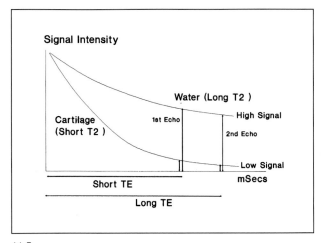

11.5

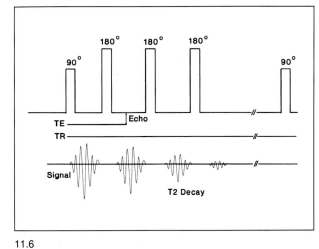

11.6

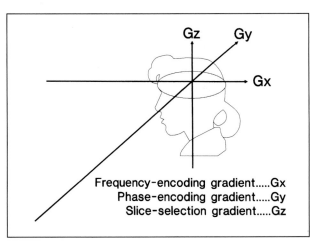

11.7

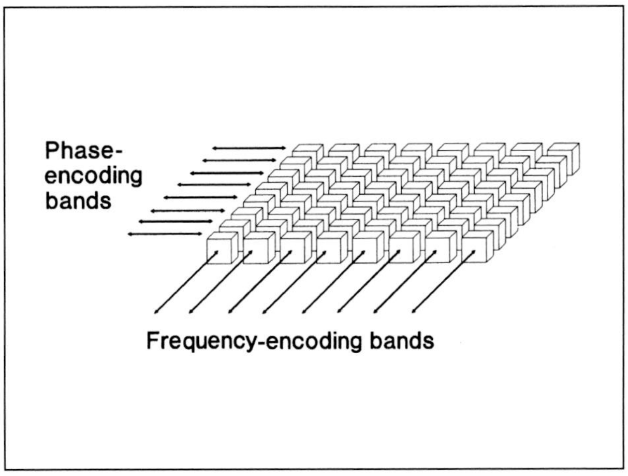

11.8

Figure **11.5**

The T2 relaxation curve is an exponential decay curve. The tissues with a short T2 relaxation time, the transverse magnetization has decayed prior to imaging. In structures with a long T2 relaxation time, the magnetization will continue to decay for a longer time (TE), hence producing bright MR signals on a T2-weighted sequence.

Figure **11.6**

Multiecho pulse sequence: TE, the time from the initial 90° radiofrequency pulse to the time the first echo signal is received; TR, the repetition time between two consecutive 90° pulses.

Figure **11.7**

Two-dimensional Fourier imaging. Spatial information is obtained by frequency encoding in the Gx plane and phase encoding in the Gy plane, following the selection of layer by the application of the Gz gradient for an axial MR scan.

Figure **11.8**

Image generation by two dimensional Fourier transformation. After slice selection, the frequency-encoding gradient is applied in one plane (x) and the layer is subdivided into bands. The phase encoding is applied in the other plane (y). The signal strength from each pixel within a frequency band is resolved by the Fourier transformation of each projection.

12

Magnetic Resonance Imaging of inflammatory conditions and tumors of the paranasal sinuses

Computed tomography (CT) and magnetic resonance imaging (MR) are the leading imaging modalities for the investigation of most disease affecting the paranasal sinuses. Benign inflammatory disease is mainly investigated by CT, MR being used as a complementary investigation in the following circumstances:

i   When CT examination has not established the diagnosis.
ii When differentiation between benign and malignant lesions is not possible by CT alone: in this event, then MR, because of its superior soft-tissue resolution, may help establish a definitive diagnosis. As MR is dependent upon the biochemical characteristics of the tissues, it can distinguish between the signal intensities of normal, inflammatory, vascular and malignant lesions. Generally speaking, all malignant lesions in the sinuses produce intermediate signal intensities (Figures 12.48, 12.50 and 12.59).
iii When multiplanar capabilities of MR imaging are useful in precisely defining tumor or inflammatory disease margins prior to treatment: this is possible without the patient having to assume any uncomfortable positions during scanning.
iv When intracranial or intraorbital extension of pathology is suspected: intracranial tumor extension and dural seeding are best demonstrated on MR because dental fillings and dense bone do not cause any artifacts (Figures 12.47–12.49). The presence of intracranial spread will alter the management of the patient.
v   When superior tumor-edge definition, soft-tissue anatomy and fascial plane delineation are required: these are far superior with MR scanning, Gd-DTPA enhanced MR scans further improve the definition of the tumor, its margins and extension into the surrounding structures (Figures 12.57).

The disadvantages of MR are the long imaging time, which may cause image degradation from motion. In addition, bone destruction and amorphous calcifications are easily overlooked on MR scans.

THE NORMAL PARANASAL SINUSES

Both CT and MR will image sinonasal mucosa. The high rate of detection of asymptomatic abnormalities of the paranasal sinuses during routine CT imaging of the head is well known. MR is far more sensitive than CT, as it detects mucosal thickening in addition to imaging changes in the nasal cavity resulting from the normal nasal cycle (Figure 12.1). The mucosa in the nasal cavity, the turbinates and the ethmoid complex are seen as low signal intensity on the T1-weighted sequence, intermediate signal intensity on the proton-density (PD) weighted sequence and hyperintense (i.e. brighter) on the T2-weighted sequence. The normal nasal cycle alternates from one side to another and is seen on T2-weighted sequences as increased brightness in the turbinates, the ethmoid sinuses and the mucosa overlying the nasal septum. As a result of the normal nasal cycle the turbinates are also larger and brighter on the side where the mucosal volume is high. This changes from one side to another during the course of the day, the cycle being anything from 1 to 6 hours. This should not be misinterpreted as inflammatory change. Up to 3 mm thickness in the sinonasal mucosa is considered to be clinically insignificant. These cyclical changes are seen only in the ethmoid sinuses and do not occur in the larger paranasal sinuses. The normal sinuses are seen as signal void cavities.

Mucosal thickening of more than 4 mm is probably pathologic, although it is not uncommon to see patients with less than 3 mm thick hyperintense mucosa who are symptomatic. The MR changes observed in the sinonasal mucosa must be correlated with the patient's clinical history and physical findings. As neither the bone nor the air within the sinuses produce signals, the demarcation between air and bone is not possible on MR scans. The major disadvantages of MR is that air, bone, calcifications and metallic densities are all seen as signal void areas, and, consequently, the subtle calcifications that characterize certain tumors can go undetected. The thin healthy mucosa may on occasion be seen as a thin layer of low signal intensity on T1-weighted sequences. The normal turbinates and the nasal septum are isointense with brain, or of intermediate signal intensity on MR sequences.

BENIGN DISEASE

Inflammation

Inflammatory changes in the paranasal sinuses can be due to a number of causes, benign and malignant. Without bony destruction, small polyps and early malignant lesion are identical on CT. Most malignant lesions evoke an inflammatory reaction in the sinonasal mucosa, thus making a carcinoma appear larger than its actual size on CT scans. With MR scans it is possible to differentiate tumor from benign inflammatory changes, due to the wide differences in their signal intensities (Figure 12.2–12.5). The precise size and the tumor margins are better delineated on MR scans because the signal intensities for inflammation and tumor are different.

Normal sinonasal mucus is a combination of secretions from the submucosal glands, and the proteinaceous secretion from the goblet cells. Transudates are serous collections with hydrogen protons in abundance. The free mobile hydrogen protons in fluids give rise to long T1 and T2 relaxation times. Consequently, the classic appearance is low signal intensity on T1-weighted scans and hyperintensity (brighter) on T2-weighted sequences. Other factors that influence the T1 and T2 relaxation times of sinus fluid are the presence of proteinaceous material, hemorrhage, the viscosity of the fluid and the temperature.

Unlike serous collections, inflammatory fluid is composed of protein-rich fluid, with a variable hydrogen proton level. This makes inflammatory fluid appear either as a bright signal on both T1-weighted and T2-weighted sequences or as a combination of low and high signal intensities.

Chronic obstruction to the ventilation and drainage pathway of a sinus results in the prolonged retention and hence accumulation of fluid. The biochemical characteristics of retained fluid secretions in the sinuses may change over a period of time. The water is slowly absorbed, resulting in thicker fluid. If the obstruction of the sinus continues, then the chronic reaction may stimulate the goblet cells of the lining epithelium to produce a fluid which is rich in protein. Histologically, goblet-cell metaplasia will be seen. As a consequence, the water is slowly absorbed and is replaced by a protein-rich secretion. This makes the fluid gelatinous, thick and viscous. As protein molecules shorten the T1 and T2 relaxation time, a proteinaceous fluid is bright or hyperintense on T1 and T2-weighted sequences. With an increase in the amount of glycoprotein production, there is an increase in the binding of the hydrogen molecules. This further reduces the amount of mobile hydrogen. The decrease in the water content further reduces the T1 relaxation motion of the glycoprotein complex results in a shorter T2 relaxation time. The pasty thick material may eventually be replaced by a dry desiccated material in the sinus lumen. As there are no remaining free mobile hydrogen protons, the substance has an extremely short spin-echo time and is seen as signal void (black) areas on T1- and T2-weighted sequences (Figures 12.6–12.9). These dynamic biochemical and physiologic changes in an obstructed sinus are the basis of the MR appearance of fluid in the various MR spin-echo sequences. MR is thus complementary to CT sinus as it characterizes the fluid by the biochemical changes taking place in the obstructed cavity.

Signal void areas may be misinterpreted as a normal sinus on MR scans if a CT scan is not available for comparison. Clotted blood, fibrotic scar, mycetomas, calcium, tooth, bone or a pocket of air can also cause a signal void area in a sinus.

Sinusitis

The classic MR appearance of benign inflammatory sinusitis is thickened mucosa of low to intermediate signal intensity on T1-weighted sequences. On proton-density weighted and T2-weighted sequences, the signal of thickened mucosa is hyperintense (brighter) (Figures 12.10–12.13). Following the administration of Gd-DTPA, there is intense enhancement of the inflamed mucosa. The high signal intensity of inflamed mucosa on T2-weighted imaging sequences helps one to differentiate active inflammation from fibrosis and/or scarring, both of which are intermediate or low signal intensity on all imaging sequences (Figures 12.14–12.21). Tumors are also intermediate in signal intensity; consequently, differentiation between tumor and fibrosis is not possible by MR. Not uncommonly, the sinus cavity is obliterated by fascia or fat, and in such instances hyperintense fat in the sinus cavity is detected on T1-weighted MR scans (Figure 12.22).

Retention cysts

Retention cysts seen in the floor of the maxillary sinus are most frequently the result of occlusion of the seromucinous glands. These are often seen in healthy and asymptomatic patients. Some patients develop these cysts close to the infraorbital nerve, and this can be symptomatic. Retention cysts are hypointense on T1-weighted, and hyperintense on T2-weighted MR sequences (Figures 12.2, 12.3, 12.23 and 12.24). Retention cysts cannot be differentiated from polyps in the sinus cavity; however, such differentiation is irrelevant, as these two entities are benign, and the treatment of the two conditions are identical. One should exercise caution in the diagnosis of benign cysts in the sphenoid sinus, as cystic pituitary gland lesions eroding through the floor of the sella may present as cystic lesions in the sphenoid sinuses (Figures 12.25 and 12.26).

Sinonasal polyposis

The clinical features and CT appearance of benign nasal polyps have been discussed in Chapter 8. The characteristic MR features of sinonasal polyposis are reflections of the rich proteinaceous and watery contents of the polyps. As a polyp ages, the number of free hydrogen protons decreases; as a result, the MR characteristics are variable. These polyps are low to intermediate in signal intensity on T1-weighted, and proton-density weighted MR sequences. The hyperintensity of polyps on T1-weighted scans is usually due to increase in the protein content or due to hemorrhage within the

polyps (Figure 12.27). The hyperintense signal on T2-weighted MR sequences is due to high water content. The signal-void septa are well demonstrated on MR scans, in which hyperintense polyps are seen in the sinus lumen (Figures 12.28 and 12.29).

Chronic longstanding polypoid lesions in the sinonasal cavity undergo biochemical changes. The water content decreases significantly, and the polyps become richer in protein. Consequently the polyps have a high signal on all imaging sequences. Thus, from the MR features, one can confidently predict if the polyps have been present for a long time. On CT scans, diffuse sinonasal polyposis, which are seen as soft-tissue densities in the lumen, may sometimes seem aggressive enough to be misdiagnosed as a malignant mass. On MR scans such masses demonstrate a variation of signal intensity, varying anywhere from hyperintense signals to signal-void areas on all imaging sequences. This MR appearance is classic for benign sinonasal polyposis (Figures 12.30–12.33). Even in the presence of erosions, the inhomogenous appearance of the lesions in all sequences characterizes their benignity (Figure 12.34).

Mucocele

By definition a mucocele is the result of prolonged obstruction of the drainage pathway of a sinus, which results in the remodeling of the sinus cavity. Mucoceles are the commonest expansile lesions seen in the paranasal sinuses. The sinuses involved in the decreasing order of frequency are the frontals, ethmoids, maxillary and the sphenoid sinuses. Mucoceles commonly present as painless masses adjacent to the superomedial margin of the orbit, with or without exophthalmos, and diplopia. Mucoceles are associated with smooth erosions of the sinus walls and expansion of the sinus. These bony changes are best demonstrated on CT scans (Figures 12.6 and 12.7) and can be easily overlooked on MR scans (Figures 12.8 and 12.9).

As mentioned earlier, the secretions in a mucocele can be serous, proteinaceous, thick and pasty, or dry and desiccated. Depending on their biochemical constituents, mucoceles can be hypo-, iso- or hyperintense or signal void on both T1- and T2-weighted sequences (Figures 12.14–12.16 and 12.35–12.39): the lower the water content, the shorter the T1 and T2 relaxation times.

Those mucoceles that are signal void on T1- and T2-weighted sequences due to their desiccated contents pose a problem because they can be easily overlooked as a normal air-filled sinus. The differentiation is done by a CT scan, which will demonstrate the desiccated material in the sinus, in addition to the expansion of the sinus by the mucocele (Figures 12.6–12.9).

A recent-onset mucocele has a high water content and is hypointense on T1-, intermediate signal on proton-density and hyperintense on T2-weighted MR sequences. The water content of a mucocele that has been present for a few months is slowly absorbed and is replaced by protein rich secretions from the seromucinous glands. This makes the mucocele intermediate in signal intensity on T1-, and hyperintense on T2-weighted MR sequences. With further loss of free and mobile hydrogen protons, and an increase in the protein content, the mucocele is hyperintense on T1- and T2-weighted MR imaging sequences. A long standing mucocele is dry and desiccated, there are no free hydrogen protons, and the mucocele is seen as a signal void cavity on T1- and T2-weighted MR scans. If the expansile nature of the mucocele is overlooked, these longstanding mucoceles can be misinterpreted as a normal sinus on MR scans, as air in a normal sinus is signal void. The other features one should look for in addition to expansion of the bony walls is the hyperintense sinus mucosa seen on T2-weighted sequences. Mucosa also enhances following Gd-DTPA administration.

Sinus hemorrhage

Hemorrhage within the paranasal sinuses usually has a higher CT number than serous fluid. Visually it is difficult to differentiate fluid from blood and thickened mucosa on CT scans. However, MR is ideal for assessing an opacified sinus.

The signal characteristics for blood varies according to the chemical form in which the blood products are present. The constituents of blood undergoes several changes. In the first step in this process, the oxyhemoglobin component of the red blood cell is converted into deoxyhemoglobin, which is subsequently oxidized to methemoglobin. The intracellular methemoglobin following red blood cell lysis becomes free methemoglobin. Hemosiderin is the final degradation product of this free methemoglobin.

The importance of these biochemical changes is that the MR characteristics of acute and chronic hemorrhage vary. Without good understanding of the differences in signal intensities one could be easily misled. Deoxyhemoglobin is hypointense on T1-weighted MR sequences and becomes more hypointense on T2-weighted sequences. If the sinus is not completely filled with blood and has residual air in it, this air aids in oxidizing the clot in the sinus. Following oxidation, the sinus contents are predominantly intracellular methemoglobin which is hyperintense on T1- and hypointense on T2-weighted sequences. Once the cells break down, the intracellular methemoglobin becomes extracellular and is hyperintense on T1- and T2-weighted sequences (Figure 12.40).

It is not uncommon to see blood in the paranasal sinuses. Blood is often associated with trauma, bleeding dyscrasias and, less frequently, with hemorrhage from benign or malignant lesions. Hemorrhage following trauma can produce an inflammatory reaction of the sinus mucosa and can be easily mistaken for sinonasal polyposis.

Fungal sinusitis

Fungal sinusitis occurs both in the otherwise healthy and in the immunocompromised population. The clinical presentation varies.

The commonest presentation is a long history of sinusitis that is not responding to medical therapy. In most cases, the diagnosis is rarely made from the clinical findings. Patients are usually investigated by a CT scan to exclude any complications from chronic sinusitis. Aspergillosis is the commonest fungal infection seen in the population at large. These fungi are commonly found in the soil, decaying fruits and vegetables. The three species responsible for sinus and respiratory infections are *Aspergillus fumigatus* (the commonest), *Aspergillosis niger*, and *Aspergillus flavus*. The sinonasal and the pulmonary forms of aspergillosis are unrelated, the pulmonary form primarily being seen in immunocompromised patients.

The noninvasive form of aspergillus sinusitis usually presents as recurring sinus infections refractory to conventional antibiotic therapy. The nasal discharge is purulent and foul smelling. Air–fluid levels are not common. With mucoperiosteal erosion, pain referred to the cheek is prominent and the routine radiographs, and CT scans may show bony destruction similar to malignancy. The invasive form of aspergillosis is a rapid destructive process. In immunocompromised patients, the symptoms may not be severe enough to seek medical attention as the immune response is poor. This further delays therapy, with grave consequences. Dissemination of fungal disease is due to vascular invasion with spread to the intracranial structures and other remote vital organs. This form of fulminant disease significantly increases the mortality and morbidity in the immunosuppressed. Irrespective of the type of fungal disease, early establishment of the diagnosis is essential as the treatment is surgical removal of the fungus balls, with debridement of the infected mucosa.

Early diagnosis is now possible with CT and MR imaging. On CT scans, fungal infections are seen as high-density concentrations in the sinonasal cavity, surrounded by some fluid (Figures 12.41 and 12.42). Reactive mucoperiosteal thickening of the sinus walls with or without bony destruction is seen. The treatment is surgical debridement, re-establishment of ventilation to the sinus and antifungal treatment. With some invasive forms of aspergillosis systemic steroid therapy is also instituted.

Areas of calcifications that are easily discerned on CT examinations are not well demonstrated on MR scans (Figure 12.41). The specimens from fungal infection are rich in iron, magnesium, calcium and manganese. These heavy metals are responsible for the increase in the CT number and the hyperdensity seen on the scans.

On MR scans, the T1-weighted sequences usually demonstrate a hypointense mass in the sinus cavity, surrounded by fluid. On protein-density weighted and T2-weighted sequences the fungus balls usually show signal-void areas, and signal intensities are lower than those seen on a T1-weighted scan. In some areas, there may be no signal, due to the calcium and other heavy metal content. Inflamed sinus mucosa is usually hyperintense (Figures 12.42–12.46). The signal-void areas are easily mistaken for normal air in the sinus cavity. Most masses and polyps on T1-weighted sequences are hypointense, but their signal intensities on T2-weighted sequences vary, thus making it possible to differentiate between benign inflammatory polyps, malignant lesions and hemorrhage. Benign polyps are hyperintense and malignant lesions are hypo- or intermediate intensity. Acute hemorrhage is hypointense on T1- and T2-weighted sequences. Subacute hemorrhage is hyperintense on T1- and T2-weighted sequences. The signal characteristics of various abnormalities are summarized in Table 12.1.

Obviously there are certain limitations to MR imaging. Teeth, calcifications and air, all easily differentiated on CT scans, produce no signals and can easily go undetected on MR scans. With further refinement in MR technique and software, it may be possible to image bone, teeth enamel and calcifications. MR will continue to play a major role in sinus imaging, especially where benign lesions, such as mucoceles or fungal infections, present as apparently aggressive and malignant lesions on CT examinations.

MALIGNANT TUMORS OF THE SINUSES

Primary tumors of the paranasal sinuses can remain confined within the sinonasal cavity for long periods of time without producing any symptoms. When patients present to the physician, it may be too late, as they are symptomatic only if there is local spread to the orbital, facial or nasal surfaces of the maxillary sinuses. Hence, these tumors have a poor prognosis, due to the rapidity of dissemination after their early asymptomatic stage. The key to the management of these tumors is early diagnosis and treatment. Early diagnosis is now possible with CT and MR. CT is superior in assessing the presence and extent of bony destruction, while MR is superior in assessing the extent of the tumor, especially when intracranial and intraorbital extension is suspected (Figure 12.47–12.49).

The commonest histologic type of malignant tumor seen in the sinuses is squamous cell carcinoma. The commonest sites, in order of frequency, are the maxillary sinus, nasal cavity, ethmoid complex, frontal sinus and sphenoid sinus (Figure 12.48–12.50). Most of these tumors are low to intermediate in signal intensity on MR imaging. The exceptions to this rule are the glandular minor salivary gland tumors, which have brighter signal intensities on T2-weighted sequences due to the high seromucinous contents. The schwannomas are also bright on T2-weighted sequences, due to the cystic degeneration that these tumors frequently undergo.

Clinical presentation and diagnostic imaging

The initial clinical symptoms may not be debilitating enough to prompt radiologic investigations. Patients often receive treatment for sinusitis, which does not

Table **12.1** Signal intensity relative to brain.[a]

Abnormalities	Appearance on T1-weighted MR scans	Appearance on T2-weighted MR scans
Sinusitis	Thick mucosa hypointense	Thick mucosa hyperintense
Retention cysts	Hypointense	Hyperintense
Polyposis	Hypointense	Hyperintense
Longstanding polyps	Variable	Variable
Mucocele		
high water content	Hypointense	Hyperintense
lower water and higher protein content	Hyperintense	Hyperintense
thick, pasty content	Hypointense	More hypointense to signal void
dessicated, dry and without mobile hydrogen	Signal void	Signal void
Hemorrhage		
acute	Hypointense	Hypointense to signal void
chronic	Hyperintense	Hyperintense
Mycetoma		
cheesy content	Hypointense or isointense	More hypointense on T2-weighted MR or signal void
dry content	Signal void	Signal void

[a]Hypointense = dark; hyperintense = bright; isointense = same intensity as brain; signal void = black; variable = hypo-, hyper- or isointense or signal void.

respond to antibiotics. The patients often fail to see the prolonged and chronic nature of their disease, which results in a further delay of the diagnosis. A high index of suspicion and further investigation of the persistent unilateral sinusitis will often enable the diagnosis to be established without further delay. Hence the proper diagnosis and management of sinonasal malignancies include:

i   a thorough clinical and endoscopic examination;
ii CT and/or MR examination, so that tumor stage can be established on the basis of tumor (T) location, size, nodal (N) spread, if any, and metastasis (M), if any;
iii postoperative follow up with CT and/or MR examinations at 6 weeks, 3 months, 6 months and yearly intervals.

The importance of imaging is to assess the extent of tumor involvement, its operability, postoperative course and define the margins for radiotherapy.

The TNM staging of tumors is used by surgeons, radiotherapists and oncologists. The radiologist's role is to assist the specialists in the precise staging of tumors.

Comparison of Computed Tomography and Magnetic Resonance of tumors

Apart from being more cost-effective, more available, and less susceptible to motion artefacts, the advantages of CT over MR are that bony destruction is best demonstrated on CT, and that calcifications that characterize certain tumors, such as chondrogenic and osteogenic tumors, are well seen on CT and may go undetected on MR scans.

The major limiting factor of CT imaging is the lack of differentiation between tumor, surrounding inflammation that the tumor may have caused and stagnant viscid sinonasal secretions that may result from inadequate drainage of the obstructed sinus. The dense bones of the skull base cause significant image degradation and loss of soft-tissue details (Figures 12.47–12.50).

As MR signals depend upon the presence of free hydrogen protons, fat has a short T1- relaxation, and is seen as bright signals on T1-weighted sequences, making the contrast in MR images superior to that in CT. Most inflammatory changes and benign polyps produce bright signal intensities on T2-weighted sequences. Malignant lesions are low to intermediate in signal intensity. This difference in signal intensities between malignant tumors and the benign inflammatory reaction that these tumors often invoke assists in delineation of the tumor margins (Figure 12.51 and 12.52).

Contrast enhancement with Gd-DTPA further improves on MR scans the definition of tumor and its margins and extension into the surrounding structures (Figure 12.57).

The disadvantages of MR are the long imaging time, resulting in image degradation due to motion and the fact that bone destruction and amorphous calcifications can be easily overlooked.

Angiofibroma

Angiofibromas are highly vascular, with a tendency to recur locally. They are seen predominantly among adolescent males. The common clinical presentations include nasal obstruction, epistaxis, recurrent sinusitis and anosmia. The tumor arises from the nasopharynx and extends intracranially or into the orbit via the pterygopalatine fossa. Superiorly, the tumor can extend into the sphenoid sinus. Anteriorly and inferiorly, the tumor can enlarge and remodel the posterior wall of the maxillary sinus. Imaging is undertaken primarily to localize the tumor and define its margins prior to treatment.

Histologically, angiofibromas are benign, unencapsulated and very vascular. They are hypointense on T1-weighted scans (Figure 12.53). On proton-density and T2-weighted sequences they are of intermediate signal intensity (Figure 12.54). Being very vascular, these tumors can exhibit a salt and peppery appearance on T2-weighted sequence due to the tumor vessels, which are seen as flow-void channels.

Esthesioneuroblastoma

These tumors arise from the olfactory mucosa and are classically located in the roof of the nasal cavity. The type of surgery to be performed on these patients depends on the precise definition of these tumor margins. Those tumors that are localized to the nasal cavity, with or without extention into the adjacent ethmoid sinuses, are approached by a lateral rhinotomy. If intracranial extension is seen on MR or CT examination, then a more radical approach, with removal of the cribriform plate and the olfactory bulb, is undertaken. Esthesioneuroblastomas are intermediate or low in signal intensity on all MR sequences. Following Gd-DTPA administration, they can enhance (Figures 12.55–12.58).

Metastasis and contiguous spread of tumor from adjacent structures

Rarely, the sinuses may be the site for metastasis. The commonest primary tumors metastasizing to the sinuses are lung cancer, renal cell carcinoma, breast cancer or melanoma. The symptoms are non-specific. The CT appearances of these tumors are similar to primary sinonasal neoplasms. Destruction of bone, with or without tumor enhancement, is the usual feature. The MR features are similar to primary tumors, with intermediate or low signal intensity on all imaging sequences.

Direct invasion into the sinuses from neighbouring structures is not uncommon. The most common tumors that directly invade the sinuses are the oropharyngeal cancers, odontogenic tumors and local skin tumors, such as basal cell carcinoma or melanoma (Figures 12.51, 12.52 and 12.59–12.62).

The odontogenic tumors are inhomogenous on T1-weighted MR sequences, and on T2-weighted MR sequences they exhibit varying signal intensities, with focal areas of hyperintensity in the tumor matrix. Another pathway for spread of tumor is perineural extension of tumors to the skull base and the underlying sinuses from primary tumors on the face and scalp.

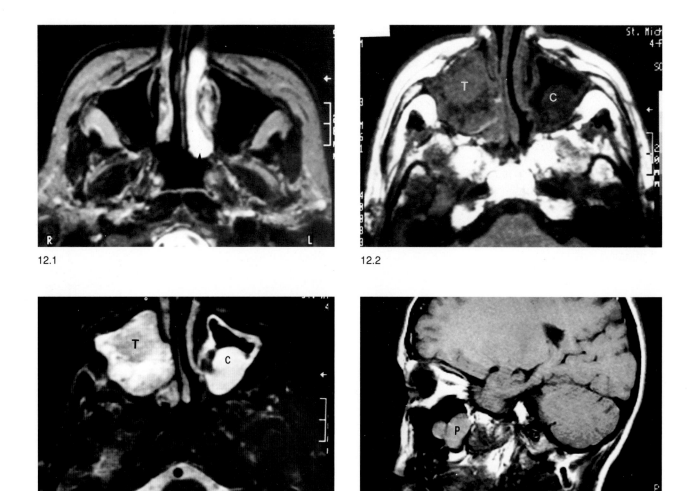

12.1

12.2

12.3

12.4

Figure **12.1**

Normal nasal cycle. This axial T2-weighted MR scan demonstrates high signal intensity in the enlarged turbinates (arrow) and nasal septum on the right side. This is the normal nasal cycle and should not be misinterpreted for an abnormality or infection.

Figure **12.2**

Malignant tumor and retention cyst. The T1-weighted MR scan in the axial plane shows the entire right maxillary sinus lumen to be filled by a mass of varying signal intensity (T). A hypointense, rounded, well-defined mass (C) is seen in the left maxillary sinus.

Figure **12.3**

Malignant tumor and retention cyst. On this T2-weighted axial MR scan the malignant tumor (T) seen in Figure 12.2 is seen to be surrounded by inflammatory hyperintense (bright) sinus mucosa. The cyst in the left maxillary sinus (C) is hyperintense, and the bright outline seen in the left maxillary sinus is the mucosal lining.

Figure **12.4**

Maxillary sinus polyp. A lobulated mass (P) in the right maxillary sinus, isointense with brain, is seen on this T1-weighted sagittal MR.

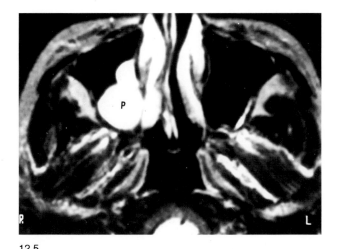

12.5

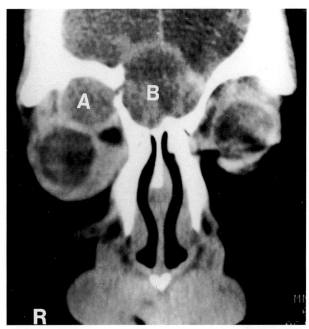

12.6

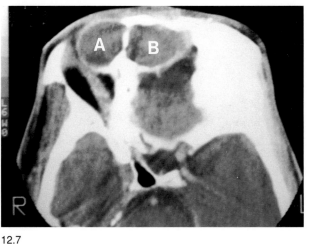

12.7

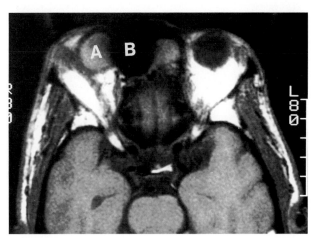

12.8

Figure **12.5**

Maxillary sinus polyp. This T2-weighted MR scan in the axial plane demonstrates the mass (P) in the right maxillary sinus in Figure 12.4 to be hyperintense.

Figure **12.6**

Frontal sinus mucocele. This patient presented with exophthalmos. The coronal CT scan demonstrates a large mucocele with smooth erosions of the bony wall, extending into the right orbit: two mucocele cavities are seen (A and B).

Figure **12.7**

Frontal sinus mucocele. The axial CT scan of the same patient as Figure 12.6 demonstrates two mucoceles (A,B) separated by a sclerotic and thickened bony septa in the frontal sinuses. The fluid collections in the two mucoceles are similar in density.

Figure **12.8**

Frontal sinus mucocele. This axial T2-weighted MR scan of the same patient as Figure 12.6 demonstrates the signal intensity of the contents of two mucoceles to be markedly different. One is isointense (A) with brain, while the contents of the other (B) are signal void.

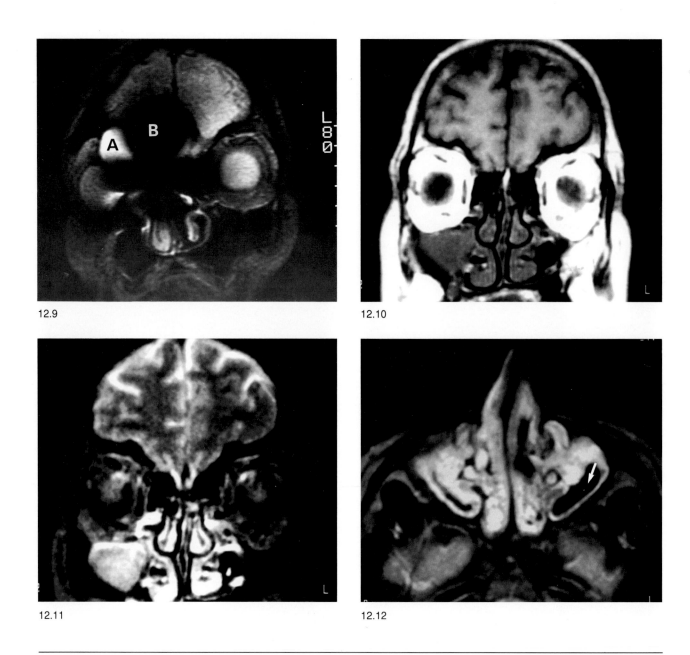

12.9

12.10

12.11

12.12

Figure **12.9**

Frontal sinus mucocele. In this T2-weighted MR scan of the same patient as Figure 12.6 the mucocele is seen as a signal void area (B). If the expansion of the sinus wall is subtle, such a mucocele can be easily overlooked on MR scans. Mucoceles have variable signal intensities depending upon their contents. Thick viscid mucoid material with few hydrogen protons will be signal void; material that has abundant hydrogen protons and is fluid will be hyperintense on T2-weighted sequences (A).

Figure **12.10**

Maxillary sinusitis. This T1-weighted MR scan shows a collection in the right maxillary sinus to be isointense with brain. A hypoplastic left maxillary sinus with ipsilateral enlargement of the nasal cavity is noted.

Figure **12.11**

Maxillary sinusitis. This T2-weighted MR scan shows hyperintense mucosa, while the fluid in the sinus cavity is not as hyperintense as water is expected to be. Longstanding obstruction of the sinuses may lead to decreased quantities of hydrogen protons.

Figure **12.12**

Chronic sinusitis. This T2-weighted MR scan shows a thickened hyperintense mucosa in the maxillary and ethmoid sinus bilaterally. The dark area is air in the diseased sinus (arrow).

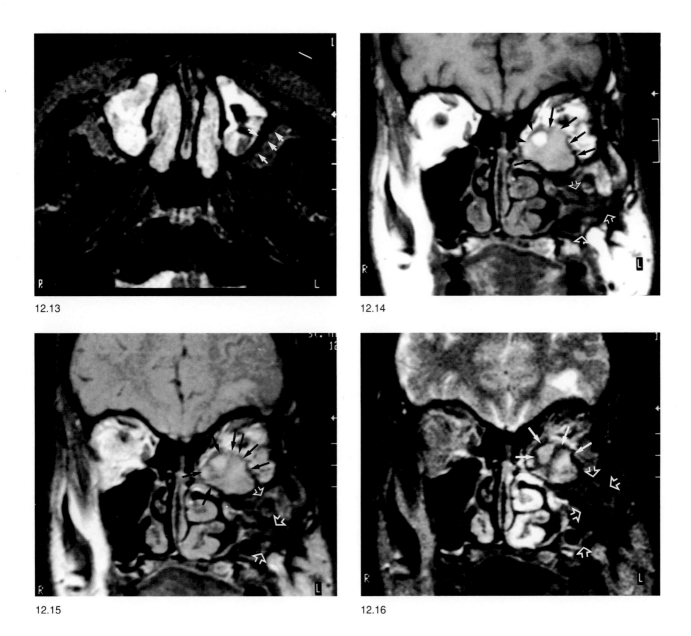

12.13

12.14

12.15

12.16

Figure **12.13**

Chronic sinusitis. Thickened and hyperintense mucosa is seen in the maxillary sinuses on this T2-weighted MR scan. Chronic reactive osteitis is seen as thickened signal void lateral maxillary sinus wall (arrows).

Figure **12.14**

Post-traumatic mucocele and scarring. This T1-weighted MR scan shows an expansile mass in the inferomedial aspect of the orbit (arrows). This patient underwent surgery for multiple fractures to the sinuses and facial bones. The left maxillary sinus lumen is replaced by linear strands of varying signal intensities (open arrows).

Figure **12.15**

Post-traumatic mucocele and scarring. The mucocele remains unchanged in signal intensity on this proton-density weighted MR scan (arrows). The scarring in the maxillary sinus appears darker (open arrows).

Figure **12.16**

Post-traumatic mucocele and scarring on a T2-weighted MR scan. A mucocele is seen as an unusual multiseptated mass (arrows) with hyperintense contents. The fibrosis and scarring (open arrows) is further reduced in signal intensity: this progressive decrease is more in keeping with scarring. Active inflammatory reaction would be hyperintense.

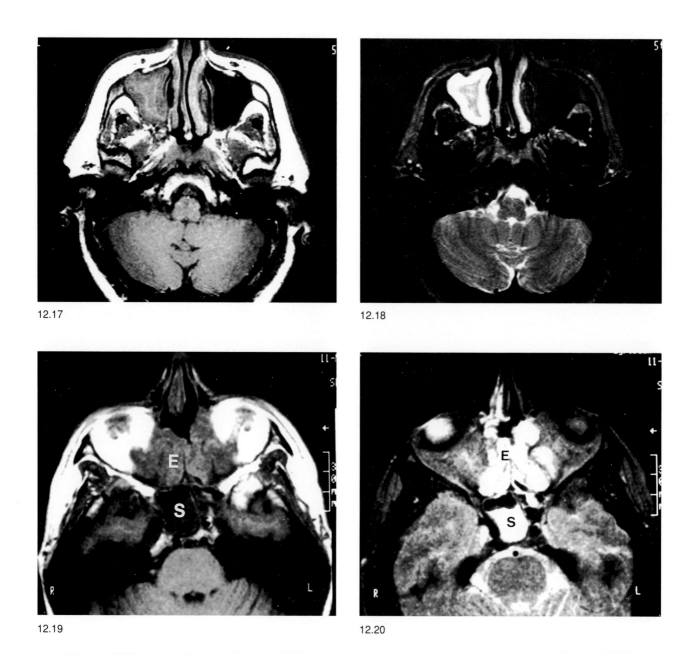

Figure **12.17**

Chronic maxillary sinusitis. On this T1-weighted MR sequence the right maxillary sinus contents are of mixed signal intensity.

Figure **12.18**

Chronic maxillary sinusitis. On this T2-weighted MR scan the right maxillary sinus mucosa is hyperintense (same patient as Figure 12.17). The fluid is of a lower signal intensity due to fewer mobile hydrogen protons. This is typical of longstanding obstruction and sinusitis.

Figure **12.19**

Ethmoid and sphenoid sinusitis. This T1-weighted MR scan demonstrates inflammatory mucosal thickening in the ethmoid sinuses (E). An air–fluid level is seen in the right sphenoid sinus (S).

Figure **12.20**

Ethmoid and sphenoid sinusitis. This T2-weighted MR scan of the same patient as Figure 12.19 demonstrates hyperintensity of the inflamed mucosa in the ethmoid sinuses (E), and fluid in the right sphenoid sinus (S) is hyperintense due to an abundance of hydrogen protons.

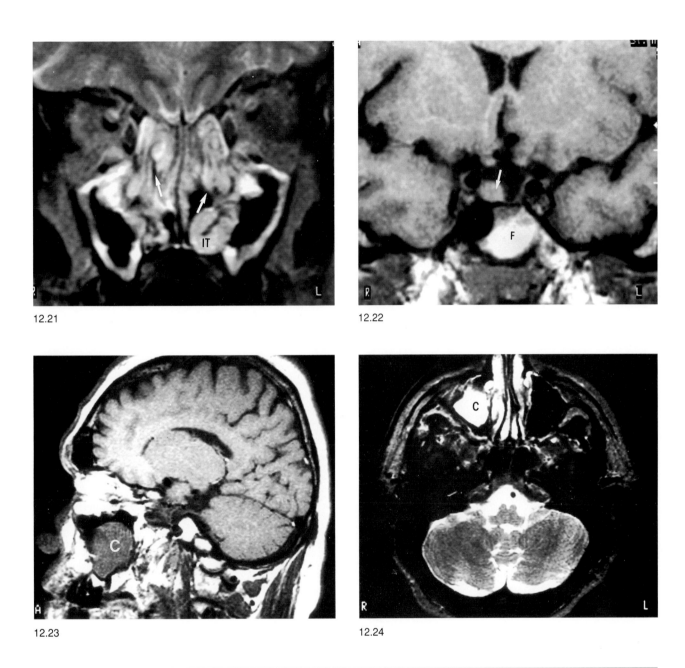

12.21

12.22

12.23

12.24

Figure **12.21**

Postoperative recurrent sinusitis. The T1-weighted MR scan (not shown) demonstrated densities in the ethmoid and maxillary sinuses to be isointense with brain. This T2-weighted MR axial scan shows hyperintensity of the thickened mucosa in the postoperative ethmoid cavity and in the maxillary sinus (arrows). These are nonspecific inflammatory changes in the ostiomeatal complex bilaterally. A large hypertrophied inferior turbinate is seen on the left side (IT).

Figure **12.22**

Postoperative changes in the sphenoid sinus. This T1-weighted MR scan shows the left sphenoid sinus lumen to be obliterated by high signal intensity fatty tissue (F) obliterating the lumen, following pituitary gland surgery. Residual pituitary tissue is seen in the sella (arrow).

Figure **12.23**

Retention cyst. A dome shaped hypointense mass in the right maxillary sinus (C) is seen.

Fig\ure **12.24**

Retention cyst. The axial T2-wighted MR scan of the cyst (C) shown on Figure 12.23 is hyperintense in signal intensity.

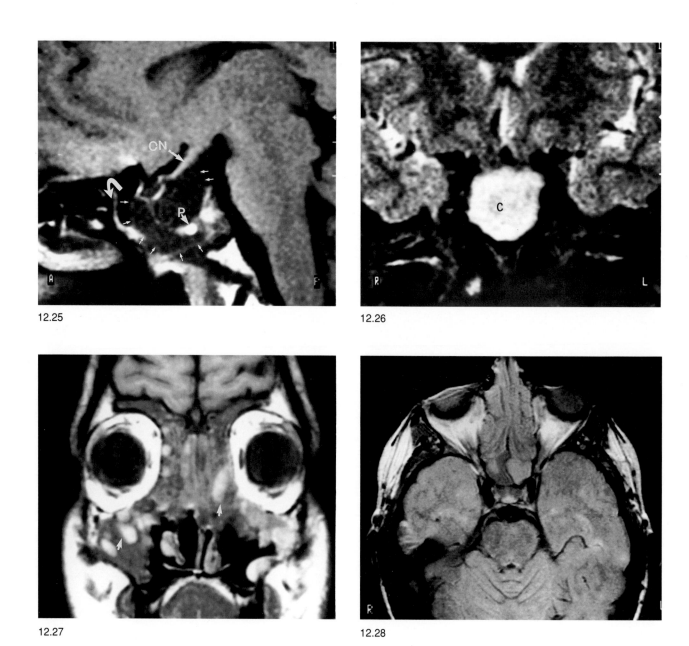

12.25

12.26

12.27

12.28

Figure **12.25**

Cystic tumor of the pituitary gland. This sagittal T1-weighted MR scan shows a multiseptated cystic mass (small arrows) arising from the gland. This cystic neoplasm has eroded through the sellar floor and fills the sphenoid sinus. Note the sinus ostium anteriorly (curved arrow), the optic nerve (ON) and high signal intensity from the posterior lobe of the pituitary gland (P).

Figure **12.26**

Pituitary tumor. On this coronal T2-weighted MR scan the cystic pituitary (C) tumor seen in Figure 12.25 fills the sphenoid sinus and is hyperintense. The roof of the sphenoid sinus is eroded. Without the clinical information, this could be mistaken for a mucocele.

Figure **12.27**

Hemorrhagic nasal polyposis. This patient had undergone several operations for massive sinonasal polyposis. This T1-weighted MR scan shows the polyps to be of varying signal intensities. The high signal intensities (arrows) seen on T1-weighted images are due to hemorrhage within polyps.

Figure **12.28**

Nasal polyposis. This axial proton-density weighted MR scan demonstrates the masses in the ethmoid sinuses to be of intermediate signal intensity. The bony septae in the ethmoid complex are well preserved.

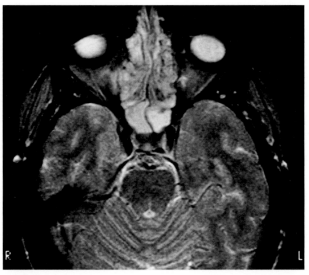

12.29

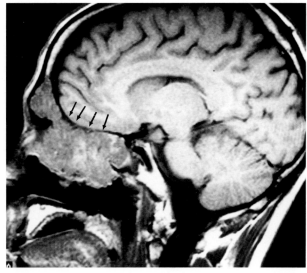

12.30

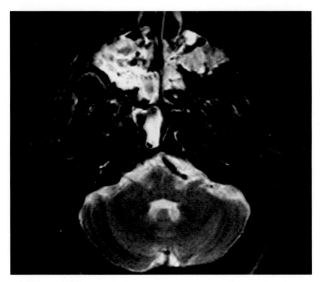

12.31

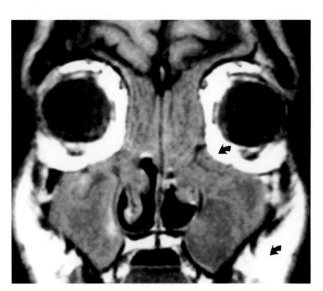

12.32

Figure **12.29**

Nasal polyposis. On this axial T2-weighted MR scan of the polyps seen in Figure 12.32, the masses are demonstrated to be hyperintense in signal intensity.

Figure **12.31**

Benign nasal polyposis. This T2-weighted MR scan in the axial plane of the same patient as Figure 12.30 demonstrates the varying signal intensities ranging from signal void to hyperintensity. This MR appearance is classic benign polyps in contrast to malignant polyps, which are of intermediate signal intensity in all imaging sequences.

Figure **12.30**

Benign nasal polyposis. This sagittal T1-weighted MR scan shows the masses in the frontal, sphenoid and the ethmoid sinuses to be of mixed signal intensity. The signal-void bone (arrows) is not eroded by the massive polyposis.

Figure **12.32**

Sinonasal polyposis. This patient underwent multiple polypectomies, and ethmoidectomy. The T1-weighted MR scan demonstrates masses of intermediate signal intensity in the maxillary and ethmoid sinuses bilaterally, with hypertelorism. The bright signals seen in the orbits and the cheeks are from the fat (black arrows).

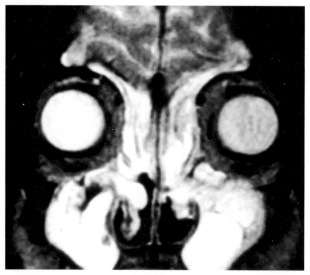

12.33

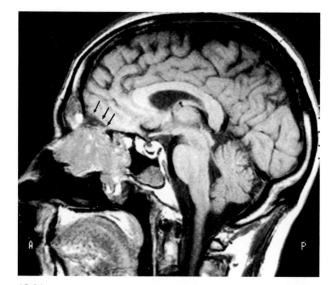

12.34

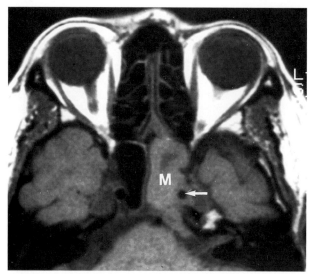

12.35

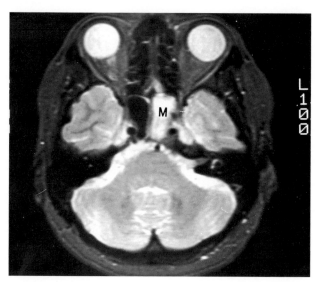

12.36

Figure **12.33**

Sinonasal polyposis. This T2-weighted scan of the same patient as Figure 12.32 demonstrates hyperintensity of the large polyps in the maxillary sinuses, and in the ethmoid complexes bilaterally.

Figure **12.35**

Mucocele of the sphenoid sinus. A mucocele of the sphenoid sinus (M) is seen as an isointense mass with a hypointense centre, surrounding the left internal carotid artery (arrow) and encroaching on to the prepontine cisterns. This T1-weighted scan defines the relationship to vital neurovascular structures.

Figure **12.34**

Sinonasal polyposis with skull-base erosion. The sagittal T1-weighted MR scan demonstrates the erosion of the skull base anteriorly (arrows) by polyps. The inhomogenous appearance of the polyps nevertheless characterizes the benign nature of this disease despite the presence of erosions.

Figure **12.36**

Mucocele of the sphenoid sinus. This T2-weighted MR scan of the same patient as Figure 12.35 demonstrates the mucocele (M) to be hyperintense due to its high water content.

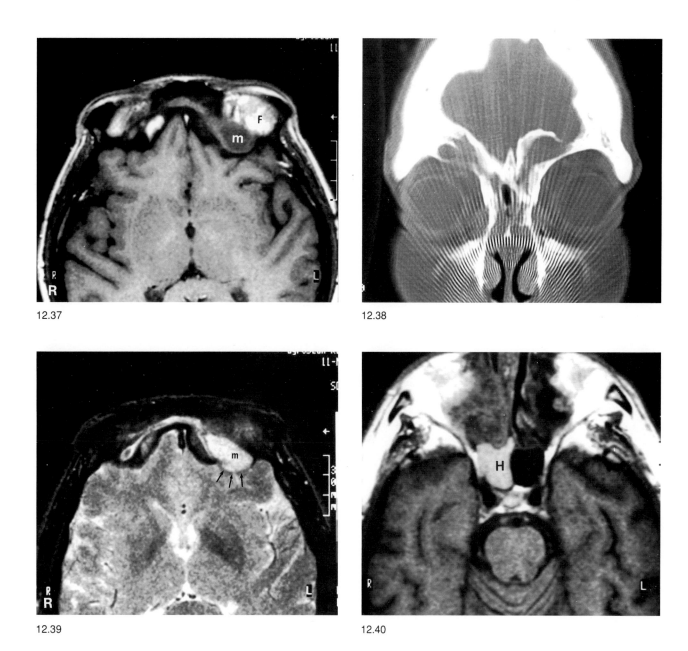

12.37

12.38

12.39

12.40

Figure **12.37**

Mucocele. This T1-weighted MR scan demonstrates high signal intensity from fat (F) and a hypointense, well-circumscribed lesion (m) posteriorly in the left frontal sinus. The patient, who had reported recurrent frontal headaches, had been referred for MR scanning after CT scanning (Figure 12.38) proved inconclusive.

Figure **12.38**

Mucocele. This coronal CT scan of the same patient as Figure 12.37 demonstrates the obliterative procedure done for frontal sinus mucoceles. The cause for recurrence of the patient's symptoms could not be ascertained from the CT scan, and MR scanning was required.

Figure **12.39**

Mucocele. This T2-weighted MR scan of the same patient as Figure 12.37 shows the mucocele (m) to be hyperintense. The posterior wall of the mucocele is eroded (arrows).

Figure **12.40**

Sinus hemorrhage. This T1-weighted MR scan demonstrates hyperintense hemorrhage (H) in the left sphenoid sinus.

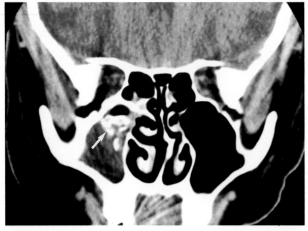

12.41

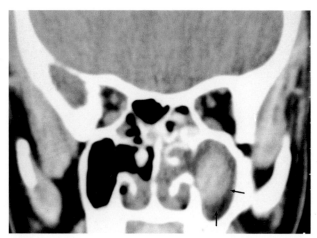

12.42

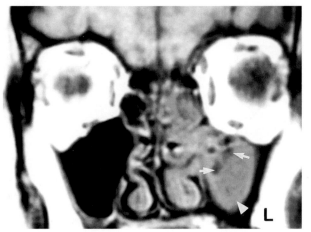

12.43

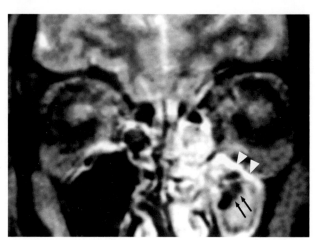

12.44

Figure **12.41**

Fungal sinusitis. This coronal CT scan demonstrates sinusitis in the left maxillary sinus, with dystrophic calcifications in the fungus ball (arrow).

Figure **12.42**

Fungal sinusitis. This coronal CT scan demonstrates a high-density mass in the left maxillary sinus, with a rim of inflamed sinus mucosa, which is low density (black arrows). The high-density mass is also seen in the ethmoid complex.

Figure **12.43**

Fungal sinusitis. This T1-weighted MR sequence of the same patient as Figure 12.41 demonstrates a signal-void area in the mass which is isointense with brain (arrows). Ferromagnetic compounds and calcium in the mycelia of the fungus cause the signal void. There is an inhomogenous increase in the signal from the inflamed sinus mucosa (arrowhead).

Figure **12.44**

Fungal sinusitis. Proton-density weighted MR scans (not shown) demonstrated further decrease in the signal intensities of the contents of the maxillary sinus. This T2-weighted MR scan shows the fungus concretions to be darker (black arrows), i.e. signal void. This is surrounded by intensely bright high signal intensity from the inflamed maxillary sinus mucosa (arrowheads).

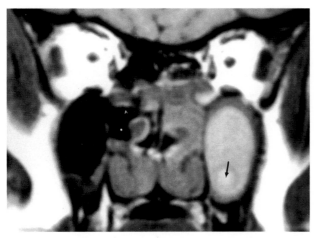

12.45

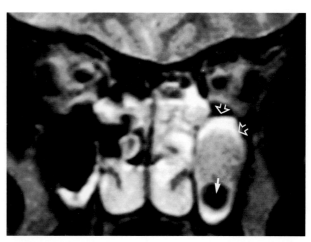

12.46

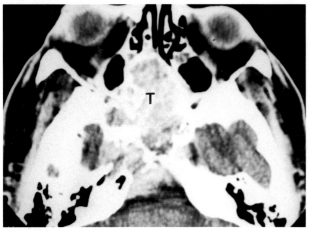

12.47

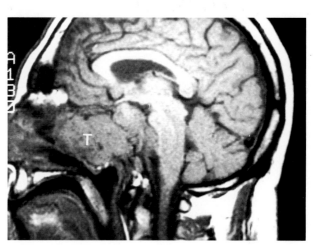

12.48

Figure **12.45**

Fungal sinusitis. This T1-weighted MR scan demonstrates a hyperintense mass in the left maxillary sinus, surrounded by hypointense fluid (arrow). A second hyperintense focus is seen in the maxillary sinus.

Figure **12.47**

Squamous cell carcinoma of the sphenoid sinus. This axial CT scan demonstrates an enhancing, destructive mass (T) eroding the sphenoid sinus and the petrous ridge. Artifacts from the dense bones of the base of the skull are seen to cause significant degradation of the image.

Figure **12.46**

Fungal sinusitis. This T2-weighted MR scan shows the hyperintense focus in the left maxillary sinus seen in Figure 12.45 as signal void (arrow). The remaining contents of the sinus are decreased in signal intensity in comparison to the T1-weighted MR scan. The inflamed sinus mucosa is hyperintense (open arrows). The proton-density weighted scan showed the maxillary contents as of lower signal intensity in comparison to the T1-weighted scan. This progressive decrease in the signal intensity on T2-weighted scans compared to T1-weighted scans is typical of fungal infection in the sinuses. Intrasinus hemorrhage can resemble fungal sinusitis: the difference is in the T2-weighted scan, where the hemorrhagic area is decreased in signal intensity, but not to the extent seen in fungal sinusitis. The inflamed sinus mucosa is hyperintense.

Figure **12.48**

Squamous cell carcinoma of the sphenoid sinus. This sagittal T1-weighted MR scan of the same patient as Figure 12.47 clearly delineates tumor (T) extension anteriorly into the ethmoid complex, with destruction and erosion of the anterior wall of the sphenoid sinus. There are no artifacts from bone on MR scans.

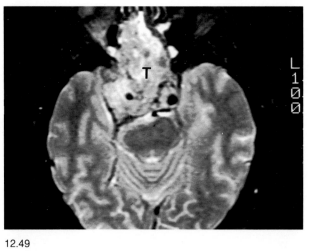

12.49

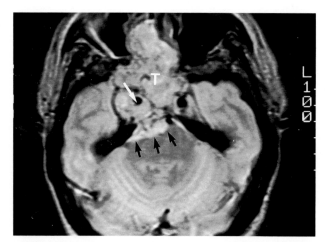

12.50

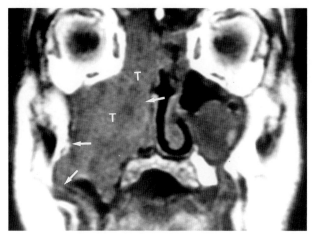

12.51

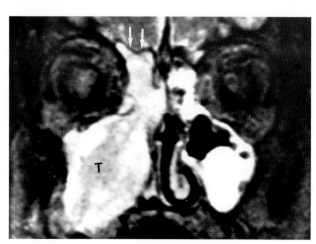

12.52

Figure **12.49**

Squamous cell carcinoma of the sphenoid sinus. This T2-weighted MR scan of the same patient as Figure 12.47 demonstrates the malignant lesion (T) to be inhomogeneous and of varying signal intensity, with focal areas of hyperintensity. The internal carotid artery is encased by the mass.

Figure **12.50**

Squamous cell carcinoma of the sphenoid sinus. This proton-density weighted sagittal MR sequence of the same patient as Figure 12.47 shows a mass of varying signal intensity arising from the sphenoid sinus. The mass (T) extends superiorly to involve the sella and encases the right internal carotid artery (arrow). Posterior extension (black arrows) into the prepontine region, with shift of the basilar artery, is well seen. As bone does not cause artifacts on MR scans, this is an excellent example of the superior soft-tissue resolution unobtainable on CT.

Figure **12.51**

Ameloblastoma. This T1-weighted MR scan shows an inhomogenous mass (lower T) of intermediate signal intensity in the right maxillary sinus, with scattered hypointense foci (necrotic areas) in the mass. The mass is seen to destroy the walls of the maxillary sinus, visualized on MR as loss of the signal void bony margins (arrows). Medially, the mass is seen to block the entire nasal cavity; superiorly, it extends (second T) into the ethmoid sinus.

Figure **12.52**

Ameloblastoma. This T2-weighted MR sequence of the same patient as Figure 12.51 shows the tumor (T) to have focal areas of hyperintensity from necrosis, surrounded by the hyperintense inflamed mucosa. A cyst is seen in the left maxillary sinus, with inflammatory changes in the left anterior ethmoid sinus. The roof of the ethmoid sinus is intact; there is no evidence of intracranial extension of tumor (arrows).

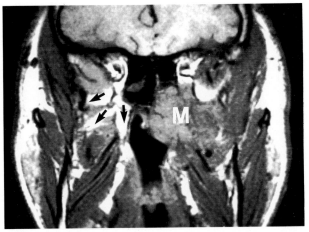

12.53

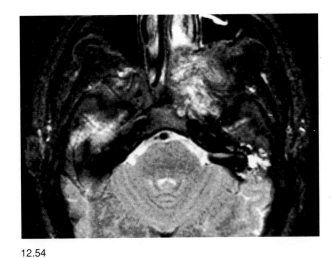

12.54

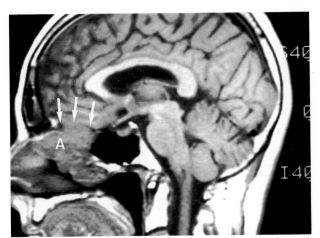

12.55

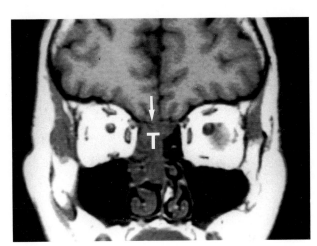

12.56

Figure **12.53**

Angiofibroma. This coronal T1-weighted MR sequence demonstrates a mass (M) isointense with brain in the nasopharynx, left ethmoid complex, and the nasal cavity. The mass extends laterally into the left pterygopalatine fossa, and the pterygoid muscles are involved. Note the normal demarkation of the muscles by the bright signals from fat on the normal side (arrows). These fatty planes are lost by tumor infiltration on the left side.

Figure **12.54**

Angiofibroma. This axial T2-weighted MR scan of the same patient as Figure 12.53 demonstrates the mass to be variable in signal intensity. The mass is seen invading the middle cranial fossa, inferior orbital fissure and cavernous sinus. The inflamed sinus mucosa is hyperintense.

Figure **12.55**

Esthesioneuroblastoma. This sagittal T1-weighted MR scan demonstrates a homogenous mass isointense with brain (A). The mass is eroding the cribriform plate (arrows) and extends outside the dura on the undersurface of the frontal lobe in the anterior cranial fossa.

Figure **12.56**

Esthesioneuroblastoma. This coronal T1-weighted MR scan of the same patient as Figure 12.55 shows the mass (T) to arise from the roof of the nasal cavity, with invasion of the ethmoid complex on the right side. The ethmoid fovea is destroyed (arrow).

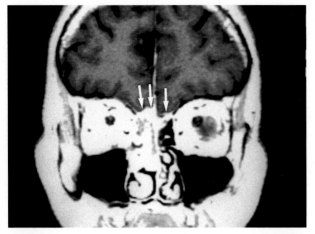

12.57

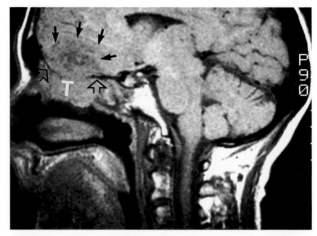

12.58

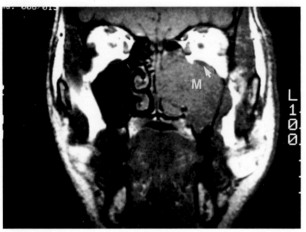

12.59

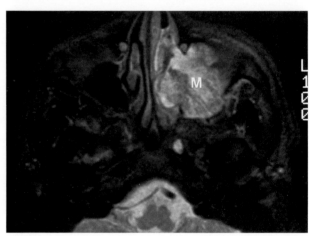

12.60

Figure **12.57**

Esthesioneuroblastoma. The Gd-DTPA enhanced MR scan of the same patient as Figure 12.55 shows enhancement of the tumor matrix, with intracranial extension and meningeal involvement (arrows). The brain is elevated by the tumor, though tumor does not infiltrate the brain.

Figure **12.58**

Esthesioneuroblastoma. This sagittal T1-weighted scan demonstrates a homogenous sinonasal mass (T) isointense with brain. This mass has destroyed the floor of the anterior cranial fossa. Although bone is not imaged on MR scans, the normal signal-void floor (open arrows) of the anterior cranial fossa is replaced by the tumor. There is direct tumor invasion into the frontal lobe (black arrows).

Figure **12.59**

Metastatic melanoma. On this T1-weighted scan a mass (M) isointense with muscle is seen in the maxillary sinus extending to involve the floor of the nasal cavity. The mass is destroying the walls of the sinus. The inferior rectus muscle is involved by the tumor mass in the orbit (arrow).

Figure **12.60**

Metastatic melanoma. On this T2-weighted scan of the same patient as Figure 12.59, the mass (M) in the maxillary sinus is of mixed signal intensity. The thin rim of hyperintensity is the inflamed sinus mucosa. There are no specific signal intensity or other features that can characterize any tumor on MR.

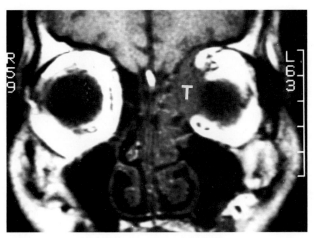

12.61

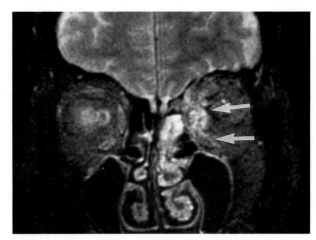

12.62

Figure **12.61**

Basal cell carcinoma. This T1-weighted MR scan demonstrates a mass (T) of intermediate signal intensity in the ethmoid sinus, destroying the lamina papyracea, with extension into the orbit.

Figure **12.62**

Basal cell carcinoma. This T2-weighted MR scan of the same patient as Figure 12.61 demonstrates the inhomogenous mass to be of varying signal intensity, with hyperintense areas in the ethmoid complex and in the medial aspect of the orbit (arrows).

13

Three-dimensional reconstruction imaging of the paranasal sinuses

Neal Lofchy   John Stevens   Judy Trogadis

Recent advances in computer technology have vastly changed the practice of medicine today. Perhaps the most striking of these have been advances in diagnostic imaging. Computed tomography (CT), magnetic resonance (MR), and positron-emission tomography (PET) scans have greatly improved diagnostic capabilities. We now, however, have the ability to convert these two-dimensional (2D) images into three-dimensional (3D) objects. In the early and mid 1980s, researchers developed the use of computer-assisted 3D reconstructions from serial electron micrographs for the study of neuronal form and function (Stevens et al. 1980, Stevens and Trogadis, 1984). More recently, clinical applications for this technology have been developed that culminated in the first 3D neuroimaging meeting at Johns Hopkins University in October of 1990 (Price and Zinreich 1989, Zinreich et al. 1990a, b). This chapter is concerned with the technique of 3D imaging and its applications in reconstruction of the paranasal sinuses.

VOLUME INVESTIGATION

The process of 3D imaging is part of a larger process termed volume investigation (VI). In order to understand VI, it is helpful to compare it with computer-assisted design (CAD). CAD uses a computer workstation to create or design new objects, whereas VI uses a workstation to convert an existing object into a 3D computer image. This image is created or reconstructed from serial 2D cross sections taken from the original object. These may be obtained nondestructively from CT, MR, and PET scans, or confocal microscopy, or destructively from light and electron microscopy or serial digitized photographs.

Volume investigation involves three basic steps: 1, reconstruction; 2, display and 3, analysis.

In a typical clinical study, a set of serial images may be obtained using nondestructive techniques such as CT or MR. For optimal accuracy, these should be adjacent cross sections with no overlap or gaps from one section to the next.

Reconstruction

The serial images used at a VI workstation are composed of a 2D array of small dots or pixels. The software of the workstation in the reconstruction process creates a 3D representation by converting each pixel into a cube of data, called a voxel. This array of voxels represents the total 3D structure of the original object.

It is important that the outline or edge of each object of interest within the voxel volume be identified. This is accomplished by a process termed segmentation (Figure 13.1). For example, bone and soft tissue can be distinguished on CT scanning as objects with differing Hounsfield densities (between 500 and 2000, and between 0 and 50, respectively). These selected densities can then be converted into groups of identified voxels. More sophisticated methods, however, are required for MR scan data as one must distinguish between objects of differing signal intensity, not density. Identifying where a surface starts and stops — whether it is by differing densities or signal intensities — is always called object segmentation. Once appropriate segmentation levels and boundaries are determined, reconstruction can begin in order to create a 3D image.

Display

Viewing of the reconstructed 3D image represents the next step. Here the object of interest can be seen as a solid rotating surface or volume, which helps in understanding its relationship to other objects, its relative size, geometric shape, etc.

Analysis

This step involves both qualitative and quantitative examination of the volumetric data. Qualitative analysis consists of detailed study of the reconstructed object using a variety of display options. Examples include rotation, magnification, light and surface texture enhancement, selective translucency, and the shaving of objects to reveal inner structure. A user can thereby interact with a VI workstation in order to more fully understand the geometric relationships within an object's volume. More objective analysis can be achieved by quantifying these relationships with volumes, distances and surface areas, as well as statistical characterization of the object itself. In this regard, quantitative analysis has proven to be of value in both scientific applications and clinical research (Stevens and Trogadis, 1990).

APPLICATIONS FOR IMAGING THE PARANASAL SINUSES

Three-dimensional images of the paranasal sinuses are reconstructed from serial CT scan slices. These slices may be axial or coronal; however axial images are preferable, to avoid inclusion of dental artifact that often obscures sinus anatomy on coronal slices. Reconstructions have been made using varying slice width intervals — accuracy, of course, increases as

slice width decreases. A slice width of 3.0 mm is adequate to provide an accurate reconstruction without undue radiation exposure to the patient. Figures 13.2–13.6 give examples of 3D scan reconstructions.

Reconstructions from serial MR slices are possible, but these will not give adequate information on bone. MR data, however, will provide superior soft-tissue resolution. This is advantageous for 3D imaging of neoplastic processes within the sinuses.

The technique of 3D imaging is proving to be beneficial for patient communication, medical education, and preoperative surgical planning. Furthermore, new technology has recently been developed to assist intraoperatively as well (Leggett et al. 1991). This so-called viewing wand is an intraoperative localization device that combines a 3D imaging workstation loaded with the patient's preoperative CT study and a hand-guided, position-sensing, articulated arm mounted on the side of the operating table. This arrangement enables correlation of the patient on the operating table with the 3D CT image, thereby providing visualization, localization, and guidance during an operative procedure. This is currently being used *in vivo* for selected neurosurgical procedures. Further development of this technology will allow for its use with functional endoscopic sinus surgery. The potential advantages include reduced risk of damage to orbital and/or intracranial structures and improved surgical training techniques.

There are inherent limitations of VI, however, that require consideration. It is a time-intensive procedure requiring a skilled technician with knowledge of radiographic anatomy — the VI process is interactive, not automated. In addition, the accuracy of the shape or calculated volume of the reconstructed 3D object is dependent upon the quality of the original 2D data. As techniques of paranasal sinus imaging improve, so will the quality of the 3D reconstructions.

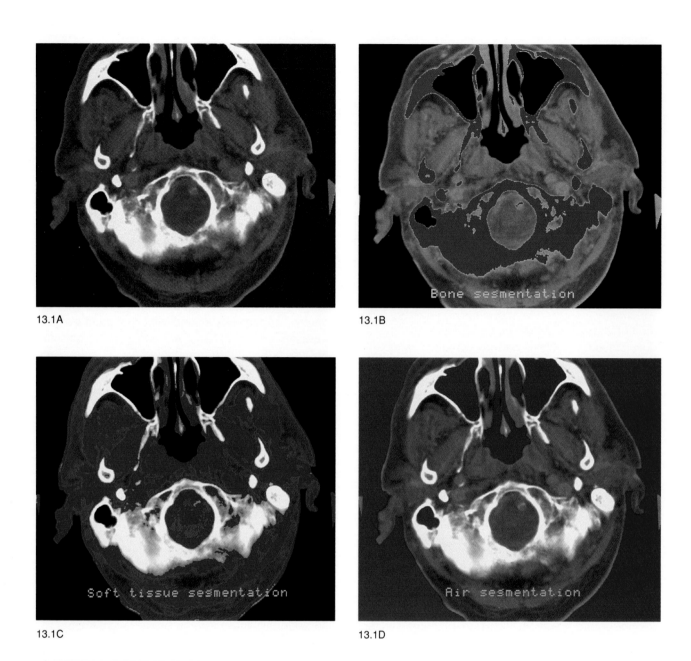

13.1A

13.1B

13.1C

13.1D

Figure **13.1**

Object segmentation of tissues of varying Hounsfield densities on an axial CT image through the maxillary sinuses. The original 2D image (A) is shown, together with segmentation for reconstruction of bone (B), soft tissue (C) and air (D).

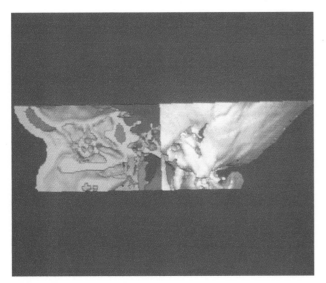

13.2

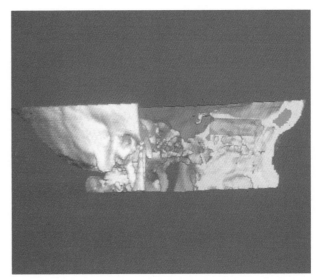

13.3

Figure **13.2**

Reconstructed lateral wall of right nasal cavity. The frontal and
sphenoid sinuses (in red) are seen as well as the semilunar
hiatus, and the middle ethmoid air cells opening onto the
ethmoid bulla.

Figure **13.3**

Reconstructed lateral wall of left nasal cavity. The bone
overlying the optic nerve (in green) has been made transparent
to demonstrate the nerve's proximity to the posterior ethmoid
cells.

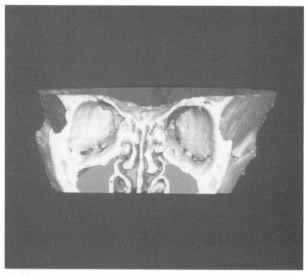

13.4A

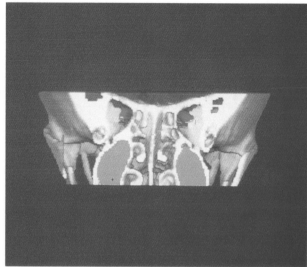

13.4B

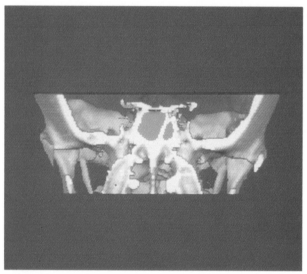

13.4C

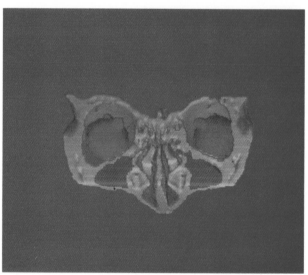

13.5

Figure **13.4**

Reconstructions with selected coronal views (A) through the maxillary antra showing the ostia bilaterally, (B) at the level of the optic nerves showing their relationship to the posterior ethmoid air cells,. and (C) through the sphenoid sinus.

Figure **13.5**

Posterobasal view of orbits and nasal cavity with globes and optic nerves (green). The maxillary sinus ostia are clearly visible.

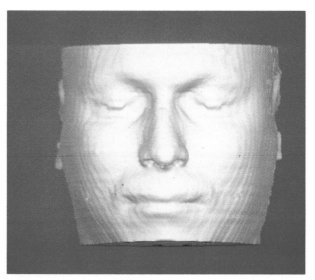

13.6A

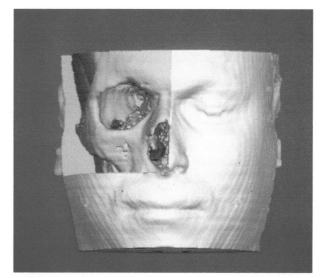

13.6B

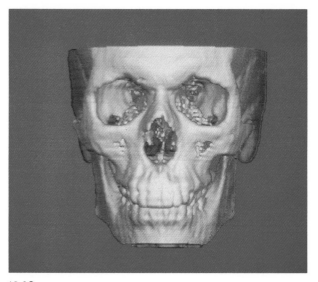

13.6C

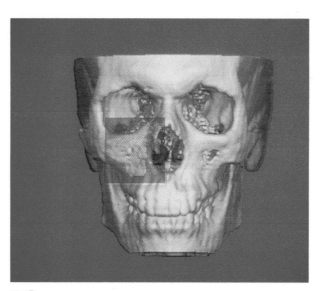

13.6D

Figure **13.6**

Three-dimensional reconstruction of a CT scan of a patient with an antral choanal polyp. (A) Overlying skin intact. (B) Skin selectively cut away to reveal underlying bone and polyp (red) within the nasal cavity. (C) Skin removed. (D) Bone overlying maxillary antrum made translucent to reveal antral portion of polyp.

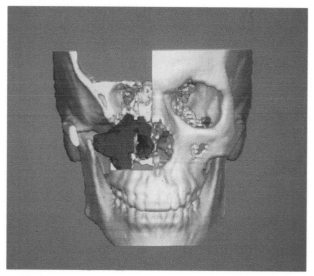

13.6E

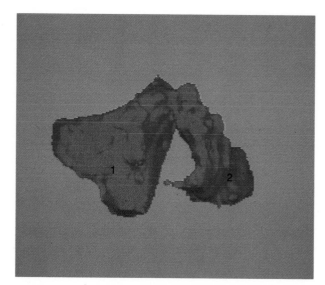

13.6F

Figure **13.6** *continued*

(E) Bony maxilla removed to display entire polyp. (F) Polyp with antral (1) and choanal (2) portions.

14

Computer-assisted surgery of the paranasal sinuses

Ludger Klimek   Ralph Mösges   Michael Hawke

Endonasal surgery has become standard for the treatment of diseases of the paranasal sinuses. The endonasal approach is no longer the exception, as there are very few diseases of the paranasal sinuses that must be treated via the external approach. This was not always the case. Ever since its introduction before the turn of the century, and up to the late 1970s, endonasal sinus procedures were considered to be extremely risky and in many hospitals were prohibited as they were felt to be too dangerous. The renaissance of these procedures arose when visual aids such as the microscope, the endoscope and magnifying glasses were introduced and used in combination with newly developed functional surgical techniques (Wigand 1981, Stammberger 1991).

Extensive statistics have proved that the complications of endonasal sinus surgery are rare and no more frequent than with the external approach. However a 2% complication rate during endonasal surgery is still widely accepted (Freedmann and Kern 1979, Wigand 1981, Stankiewics 1989, Rauchfuss 1990). The complications are: orbitoocular, vascular and encephalomeningeal. The reasons for the residual complication rate are often found in a lack of intraoperative orientation. When paranasal sinus procedures are carried out endonasally, orientation is often reduced by bleeding, with a resulting impairment of the surgeon's field of view. Moreover, procedures that rely on topographic landmarks are less precise when previous surgical procedures or tumor have destroyed these landmarks.

The objective of the computer-assisted surgical system presented in this chapter is to reduce the rate of complications by improving the surgeon's intraoperative orientation. The prerequisite of preventing the surgeon from violating critical structures is the necessity to indicate at any given time the topographic relationship between the instrument and the vulnerable structures.

THE COMPUTER-ASSISTED SURGERY SYSTEM

The computer-assisted surgery (CAS) system described here was assembled from existing and newly developed hardware in collaboration with the Institute for Measuring Techniques, and the Department of Otorhinolaryngology, Plastic, Head and Neck Surgery, Aachen Technical University (RWTH), Aachen, Germany, from 1984 to 1987 (Schlöndorff et al 1987, Mösges and Schlöndorff 1988, Mösges et al 1989, Adams et al 1990). The CAS system has been shown to be extremely helpful as an orientation aid in skull-base surgery, orbital surgery and neurosurgical procedures (Mösges and Schlöndorff 1988, Klimek et al 1991a,b, Laborde et al, in press). CAS has since been further developed and adapted to the special requirements of paranasal sinus surgery. The system consists of three components: an image generation device, image processing equipment and a location measuring system (Figure 14.1).

Image generation

For image generation a tomographic imaging system, either computed tomography (CT) or magnetic resonance imaging (MR) is required. At our hospital the computer tomographs Somatom 2, Somatom DR or Somatom Plus, or a magnetic resonance tomograph Magnetom (Siemens, Germany) are available. For paranasal sinus surgery, CT scans utilize 1 or 2 mm thick transverse (axial) cuts that are continuous and non-overlapping slices are taken (approximately 30–60 slices). Axial cuts are taken primarily for the avoidance of dental artifacts. The data are then transmitted either by floppy disks or via a fiberoptic network, the transportation medium of the experimental PACS (Picture Archiving and Communication System) of Aachen University Hospital.

Image processing

A specially developed workstation is used for the creation of the three-dimensional model and for further image processing. The computer system currently employed is based on the VME-bus. The central processing unit (CPU) module is an Eltee R Eurocom-5-R equipped with a MC 68020 processor and 68681 coprocessor. The most important task of the CPU is the generation of the voxel model and the transformation of the co-ordinates of the 3D co-ordinate digitizer. 360 and 80 MB hard disks are used for mass storage. The memory capacity is sufficient for the storage of 128 CT or MR images. As usual, the images are displayed in grey shades, whereas graphic and alphanumeric information — such as the co-ordinate digitizer's position or pull-down menus — are superimposed in arbitrary colors via a color 'look-up' table. For the display of the 3D model, special hardware has been developed: the 3D co-ordinate transformer. It takes only 90 ms for the visualization of a 512² image, independent of the specific transformation coefficients (angle of the sectional views, zoom factors, etc.) Either a pseudo-plastic 3D image can be produced or the examiner can look into the area from all sides and in all layers by moving an electronic 'mouse'. Visualization of three perpendicular slices (sagittal, coronal, axial) is standard (Figure 14.2).

Three-dimensional co-ordinate measurement

Electromechanical 3D co-ordinate digitizers have been developed for applications in mechanical engineering. The individual arm segments of these devices are connected to each other through rotary joints. The angles of each of the rotary joints is measured by rotary encoders so that the co-ordinates of the tip of a measuring probe mounted to the arm can be calculated. Such an electromechanical measuring device has been developed by our group (Figure 14.3). It has six rotary joints

and counterbalanced arm elements. We have applied optical increment encoders for shaft angle measurement. A dedicated 68008 microcomputer calculates the position of the tip of the stylus from the measured angles and the given arm lengths.

Applications in intraoperative localization

For practical application, a preoperative high-resolution CT or MRI scan is carried out. To correlate the co-ordinate system of the created 3D model with the actual position of the patient's skull relative to the measuring arm, four reference points must be defined (Figure 14.4). These markers must be visible on the CT images and also be identifiable during the operation. We use radiopaque plastic markers for this purpose. The markers are attached to the patient's skull for imaging and replaced afterwards with color markings. The co-ordinates of the markers are entered into the computer by touching them with an electronic 'mouse'.

The system must be calibrated at the beginning of the operation. This is achieved by tipping the markings with the stylus within 15 s. This procedure must be repeated after every displacement of the skull during surgery.

After the calibration procedure, the position of the instrument in the region of interest and its presentation on the screen are visually tied together; that is, the display image dynamically moves to the corresponding three perpendicular sectional views of the voxel model respective to the chosen cut in the 3D presentation. In this way, the surgeon gets precise orientation instantaneously, at a rate of 20 slices/s determined by the motion of the digitizer.

The accuracy with which instruments can be positioned with the CAS system was first determined by *in vitro* measurements. In the laboratory, the inaccuracy proved to be within 0.4 mm in a measuring volume of 0.36 m³. The accuracy of measurement with the CAS system decreases if instruments that are too thin, and thereby too flexible, are used. Additionally, we determined the accuracy for bone using a phantom skull furnished with the customary CAS markers. A study of 128 sequential CT slices with 1 mm slice thickness and 1 mm intervals was carried out and stored in the CAS system. Different measuring probes were introduced into the skull and the position of the instrument as indicated on the CAS monitor was compared with the actual position of the probe inside the skull. Measurements were repeated 80 times for each instrument. The standard deviation was 0.6 mm. In less than 15% of the measurements, the deviation exceeded voxel size of 1 mm. During intraoperative applications, soft-tissue deviations and incorrect registration of the measuring points may decrease accuracy.

CAS can be used alone or as an addition to visual aids such as the endoscope and the microscope. For use in endoscopic paranasal sinus surgery, two different methods of application are available. With the first method, the position of the endoscope itself is exactly determined with the help of CAS. For this application the endoscopes are fitted into special mounts and the established dimension data of several endoscopes are integrated into the CAS software, so that every single endoscope can be used as a measuring instrument of the CAS system. To date, the hardware and software components available allow combination of CAS with rigid endoscopes of 2.7 and 4.0 mm in diameter (Karl Storz, Endoscopy America Inc., Kennesaw, GA, USA). The surgeon looks through the endoscope at questionable structures and can display cuts at a given distance behind these structures on the monitor. This provides the surgeon with a method for looking ahead of i.e. beyond surfaces; this is especially helpful when opening ethmoid cells near the skull base.

In the second method, a measuring probe is used in addition to an endoscope (Figure 14.5). The surgeon points the measuring probe at questionable structures and compares the endoscopic appearance with the image displayed on the CAS monitor. This second technique also allows the CAS system to be used with the operating microscope.

Interactive planning of surgery on the monitor

Another advantage of the CAS system is that it allows the surgeon to call up optical views of the operating field preoperatively. With the electronic 'mouse' one can move in all directions back and forth through the CT slices, and the additionally produced image reconstructions as if walking through a corridor. These dynamics allow excellent orientation and have proven to be of assistance in the simulation of operations on the monitor. The advantages of the CAS system in operation planning lie in its real-time behavior, that is to say in the

possibility to turn objects, by means of movements of the 'mouse' in split seconds on the monitor, as the surgeon moves the patient during paranasal sinus surgery to improve the view.

Besides this easily operated basic function, special options are available which expand the applications of the system. First, using the zoom function the user can have optional details enlarged on the monitor. Small pathologies are represented more clearly, and critical regions can be examined more exactly. Second, a detailed differentiation of soft tissue becomes possible by the selection of the Hounsfield scale. The Hounsfield unit is the measure of density for CT and encompasses densities from −1000 to +3000, including all clinically relevant tissues. The density values are represented as varying shades of gray on a CT image: the CT can display 4000 different shades of gray, whilst the human eye can distinguish only about 30. Therefore, the observer would see approximately 100 adjacent density values as only a single shade and would be unable to differentiate structures in areas in which tissues differ by only a few Hounsfield units. To overcome this problem, the raw image data is selected by the radiologist for a special tissue window. Structures of interest to the examiner can so be displayed as visually distinguishable shades of gray. In general the radiologist, not the surgeon is responsible for this selection procedure. The surgeon normally receives film copies and has no possibility of tissue selection of his own. As a result, the major part of the raw CT image information is lost. With the help of a CAS workstation, surgeons can use the whole information to obtain better tissue differentiation.

THE COMPUTER-ASSISTED SURGERY SYSTEM IN PRACTICE

The Aachen CAS-system has been used for surgical purposes of the paranasal sinuses in 193 cases by 11 surgeons in five hospitals. In our department, 127 cases of endonasal procedures have been documented (Figure 14.6). Surgeons report that the localizing aid in all cases functioned exactly as soon as calibration procedures had been carried out. Intraoperative *in situ* deviation never exceeded pixel quantification of the CT scan (1–2 mm). For surgery of infectious disease, the system was used whenever more than just the maxillary sinus was affected. In agreement with Stammberger (1991) the surgeon's main interest focused on the restoration of the normal anatomy of the ethmoid sinus. In most cases, ventilation of the ethmoid was carried out. Some surgeons have however used the CAS system for radical surgery of the paranasal sinuses. In cases of disease of the sphenoid sinus, it has been ventilated and drained using a transethmoid approach (Figure 14.7). Also the frontal sinus has been approached via the ethmoid under CAS conditions. This has meant that surgeons could refrain from the time-consuming exposure of topographic landmarks. The duration of surgery also decreased dramatically.

POTENTIAL FOR THE FUTURE

Endonasal surgery in the vulnerable regions near the skull base require a safe and precise surgical technique. Most complications occur when the surgeon is not aware of the exact position of his instruments. Orbital complications have been described due to injuries to the lamina papyracea, the orbital muscles or the optic nerve itself. The optic nerve is at the greatest risk in the posterior ethmoid and sphenoid sinus. Another severe condition can occur if the anterior ethmoid artery is severed and the vessel retracts into the orbit, producing a massive orbital hematoma with compression of the globe and the optic nerve. This may result in immediate blindness if decompression cannot be achieved under emergency conditions. Damage to the internal carotid artery is a potential fatal complication that may occur from direct injury to the artery within the sphenoid sinus; it may also occur when massively pneumatized Onodi's cells are present, and the internal carotid artery bulges into these posterior ethmoid air cells and is injured in this region. Encephalomeningeal complications most often occur when missing landmarks render orientation difficult.

A typical indication for the use of the CAS system is in patients with massive nasal polyposis who have undergone previous operations and in whom the anatomic landmarks are absent, due to either the disease itself or the previous operation(s). The anatomy in the ethmoid region can be extremely difficult to identify in these cases because of extensive scarring and many adhesions. The insertion of the middle turbinate, which is an important landmark in this region, is often missing because turbinectomy was part of the previous radical surgery. The dura then is often injured at its typical weak point, the roof of the ethmoid near the exit of the anterior ethmoid artery through the cribriform plate (Stammberger, 1991). The missed diagnosis of a cerebrospinal fluid leak can result in life-threatening conditions such as meningitis or brain abscess. In clinical trials, none of the above described major complications have occurred. A solution for the problem of intraoperative localization was found in combining the preoperatively generated image data with a sophisticated 3D co-ordinate measuring device and modern computer graphics. Similar devices have been described by several authors for navigation in neurosurgery, using either electromechanical (Watanabe et al 1987, 1989, Kosugi et al 1988, Mösges and Schlöndorff 1988, Reinhard et al 1988, Mösges et al 1989, Guthrie and Adler 1991, Laborde et al in press) or ultrasonic co-ordinate measuring systems (Roberts et al 1986, Friets et al 1989, Zweifel et al 1990). These freehand navigation systems are quite different from automated surgery robots (Young 1987, Kwoh et al 1988, Drake et al 1991).

We feel, that interactive frameless devices such as the one developed by our group can fill the special needs of paranasal sinus surgery in a highly effective manner. As well as on-line localization assistance within the operation, CAS provides the surgeon with valuable information for presurgical planning. Although the number of cases is not yet sufficient for statistical analysis, we have observed that CAS enables the surgeon to avoid major complications by providing highly accurate information of the location of surgical instruments. In addition to safer surgery, the thoroughness of the procedure may be increased, especially in ethmoid surgery where overlooked diseased ethmoid cells or fissures may be the reason for persistent or recurring problems (Stammberger 1991). CAS enables the surgeon to overcome the difficulties that occur during practically every intervention when the view is reduced by bleeding or pathologies. Based upon an individual model of the patient's anatomy, the surgeon can be guided through this extremely vulnerable part of the body. Complication rates of 2% or more are no longer tolerable. The CAS systems lead the way towards a zero complication rate in endonasal surgery.

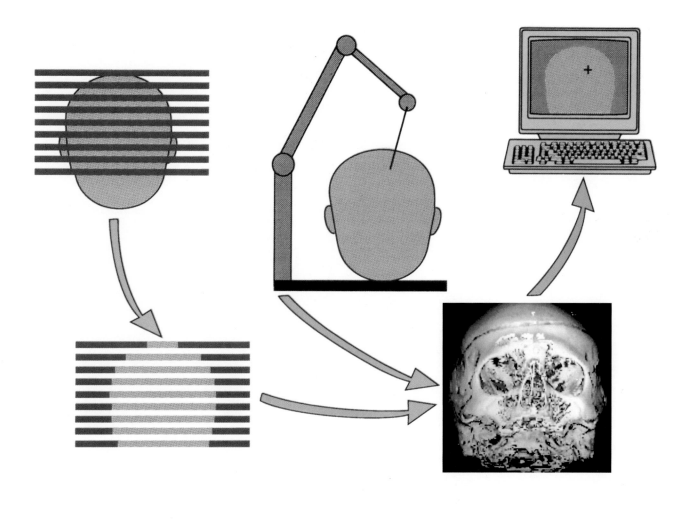

Figure **14.1**

Principles of the CAS device.

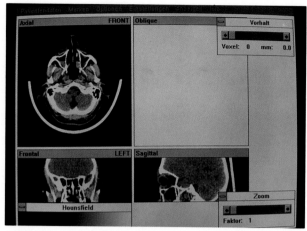

14.2

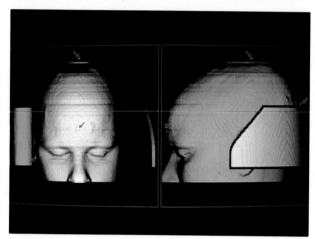

14.4

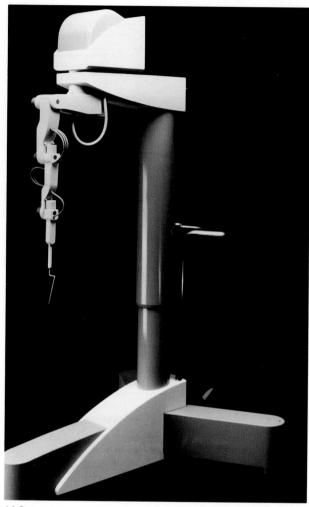

14.3

Figure **14.2**

Standard CAS display showing three perpendicular views (sagittal, coronal, axial) of the sinus.

Figure **14.4**

Display of reference markers as visualized on the CAS monitor screen.

Figure **14.3**

The electromechanical measuring arm (co-ordinate digitalizer).

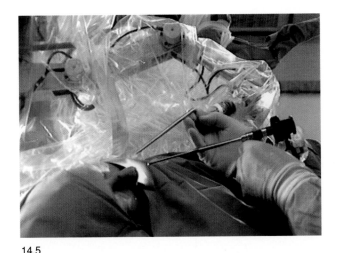

14.5

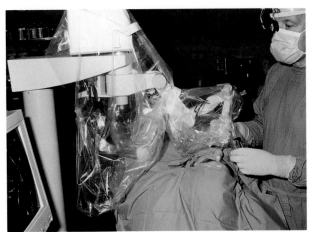

14.6

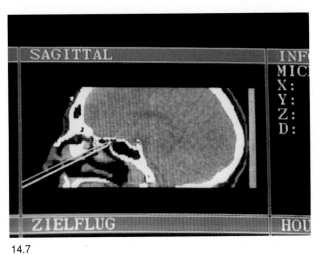

14.7

Figure **14.5**

Combination of CAS and endoscope for endonasal procedures.

Figure **14.6**

Intraoperative scenario using CAS in endonasal and paranasal surgery.

Figure **14.7**

Display of instrument position during endonasal surgery.

15

The ostiomeatal unit in childhood

Sunil Ummat   Michael Riding   David Kirkpatrick

The techniques of intranasal endoscopic and microscopic sinus surgery have introduced new tools to the armamentarium for the treatment of sinus disease, in which the role of sinus surgery has shifted in emphasis towards functional preservation and restoration. A renewed interest in the anatomy and radiologic appearance of the paranasal sinuses has arisen from the advent of these techniques.

Recurrent chronic sinusitis is a common problem in the pediatric patient population. Although the majority of patients will respond to medical management, some may require further intervention. Recently, functional endoscopic sinus surgery has been utilized for treatment of pediatric sinus disease. When operating upon children, the sinus surgeon must be aware of the differences between adult and pediatric sinus anatomy; consequently, knowledge of the developmental anatomy of the paranasal sinuses is a prerequisite for safe endoscopic and microscopic sinus surgery in children.

The ostiomeatal unit is now considered to be the critical area involved in the pathogenesis of the sinus disease. Efflux of secretions from the ethmoid, maxillary and frontal sinuses enter this region *en route* to the posterior nasal cavity. When one contemplates the development of the paranasal sinuses, the frontal, maxillary and sphenoid sinuses are those that are commonly discussed. Unfortunately, however, little information is available on the development of the ostiomeatal complex through childhood. In response to this, we commenced a study utilizing a CT scanner to chart the anatomy and development of the ostiomeatal unit area in childhood, from the age of 1 to 16 years. The emphasis was on obtaining information that would be of use to the endoscopic sinus surgeon. Furthermore, an attempt was made to obtain a set of normal values that could be of use in future comparative studies on diseased patients.

Ideally, a longer study, looking prospectively at the development of the ostiomeatal complex by following a group of patients over time with successive CT scanning, could be done. This however would be cost-prohibitive and result in unnecessary radiation exposure to children. Our study utilized existing scans for data acquisition. The use of the computer allowed the magnification of images and greater accuracy in measurement.

METHODS USED IN THE STUDY

We reviewed 196 pediatric CT scans. The children's ages ranged from 1–16 years. Patients with coronal scans, no or minimal sinus disease, and adequate anatomic resolution for measurement were included in the study. Patients with facial deformity, tumor involvement of the paranasal sinuses, growth delay or obscured anatomic detail were excluded. Ninety-six patients met the criteria and were further studied.

All patients had previously undergone CT scanning on a GE 9800 Quick scanner, utilizing a high spatial resolution program on a field of 120 × 120 mm, displayed with a 512 × 512 matrix. The collimation of the beam was 3 mm, using 120–140 kV and 40 mA.

Digital radiography to obtain a scout film was done in all cases. The coronal scans were done in the standard position for the evaluation of the ostiomeatal complex. Bone algorithms and bone windows were used for the coronal scans.

The patients were divided into groups of 1-year intervals as shown in Table 15.1. The measurements were done utilizing images generated by the computer. The images were displayed, magnified and subsequently analyzed using cursor placement. Each side was measured. The scans were randomized for age. Results were analyzed statistically using Student's *t*-test with unpaired samples.

Table 15.1 The number of patients studied in each category

Age	n
1–2	6
2–3	6
3–4	5
4–5	6
5–6	7
6–7	5
7–8	7
8–9	7
9–10	7
10–11	6
11–12	7
12–13	6
13–14	8
14–15	7
15–16	6

DIMENSIONS OF THE OSTEOMEATAL UNIT

Distance between right and left lamina papyraceae

This measurement was taken at the level of ethmoid bulla, and coinciding with a line drawn through the orbits at their midpoint (Figure 15.1A). The line represents the upper limit of the ostiomeatal complex. The results shown in Figure 15.1B and C are the mean distances throughout the various age categories. The mean ranged from 1.70 to 2.44 cm. The tabulated results can be plotted as shown in Figure 15.1C. The slope of the curve suggests a linear change.

Anterior and posterior ethmoid system widths

In measuring the anterior ethmoid system width, each side was measured separately, as shown in Figure 15.2A. The results shown here are mean distances of one side from 1 to 16 years. The means ranged from 0.39 to 0.79 cm. This represents a doubling in size. When depicted graphically, these results also suggest a linear rate of change (Figure 15.2C).

The width of each side of the posterior ethmoid system was measured separately, as shown in Figure 15.3A. The mean distance ranged from 0.48 to 1.10 cm. This increase is slightly more than that seen in the anterior system. The plotted results also depict a linear rate of change (Figure 15.3B).

It appears, then that the ethmoid cell system enlarges through childhood. There is approximately a twofold increase in width of this system, with a slighter greater increase in the posterior cells. Most endoscopes and forceps currently in use are 3 mm or greater in width. Our results suggest that further care must be taken in smaller children because of the decreased width and reduced margin of error.

Infundibular length

The infundibular length was measured as shown in Figure 15.4A. There appeared to be a greater variability in the means. This finding is best shown on a graph, through which a trend line is drawn (Figure 15.4B). The trend line shows an upward slope. The maxillary ostia open at different areas along the semilunar hiatus, and this may explain the results seen.

Infundibular width

The infundibular width measurement was found to be surprisingly constant through childhood. This measurement was taken at the entrance of the maxillary portion of the infundibulum (Figure 15.5A); at this location, it remained at about 0.2 cm ($P < 0.001$). This suggests that there may be a minimum width required for mucus flow. Infundibular width measurements were also taken further up along the infundibulum where the range was from 0.09 to 0.15 cm. The maxillary inlet gives a constant point of reference, which is why measurements were taken at this level.

The uncinate angle

The uncinate angle was measured as shown in the CT scan in Figure 15.6A. The angle was determined by the point of contact between the uncinate process and the lateral nasal wall at the origin of the inferior turbinate. Again the results (Figure 15.6B and C) showed very little change of this parameter through childhood ($P<0.001$), although there does appear to be a slight decrease in the angle through childhood.

Distance between the inferior turbinate and cribriform plate

In order to better appreciate the change of the ostiomeatal unit area in relation to the roof of the nasal cavity, the distance between the inferior turbinate and the cribriform plate was measured (Figure 15.7A). The mean distances ranged from 1.76 to 2.58 cm. We can see that there is an initial steady change in this distance, followed by a plateau during the later childhood years (Figure 15.7B). This measurement additionally conveys an estimate of the distance superiorly that is present when one is working at the level of the base of the uncinate.

Distance from the anterior nasal spine to the ethmoid roof

The nasal spine is a landmark for various anatomic measurements. Studies of cadavers and skulls have frequently used the anterior nasal spine as a point of reference. Calhoun et al (1990) have measured the distance from the anterior spine to the ethmoid foreola and the miduncinate process. The means were found to be 5.0 and 3.6 cm respectively. The mean angle from the nasal floor to the mid uncinate process was 50°. The mean angle from the nasal floor to the fovea was reported to be 62°. We computed a distance from the nasal spine to the ethmoid roof at a constant angle of 55° (Figure 15.9A). We found that in smaller children, 62° was too large an angle and the line of trajectory would land much more anterior than in older children; 55° was a more suitable angle for measurement.

Using the scout film generated by the computer, the distance from the anterior nasal spine to the ethmoid roof was measured, at a constant angle of 55° (Figure 15.8A). The range of mean distances varied from 3.38 to 5.52 cm. The data show a gradual increase throughout the early childhood years, with a plateau over the age of 10 years (Figure 15.8C).

The reults show that the distance from the anterior spine to the miduncinate process in adults is virtually the same as the distance from the anterior spine to the ethmoid roof in a child over 10 years of age. Again a guideline may be established by the data obtained in this study.

Anatomic variants

Haller's cells

We found a high incidence of Haller's cells (Figure 15.9A) in the pediatric age group. The presence of Haller's cells was found to be 79/96 or 82%. The cells ranged in size from 0.22 to 0.52 cm in width. When present, Haller's cells compose a portion of the lateral infundibular wall. In the CT scans we examined, the cells did not appear to appreciably alter the infundibular width.

This increased prevalence of Haller's cells in children is an interesting finding. The Haller's cell is situated in the lateral wall of the infundibulum and contributes to its shape. The presence of these cells did not appear to result in narrowing of the infundibulum. The information, along with the finding that the infundibular width remains similar throughout childhood, suggests that there are factors which affect the growth of the ostiomeatal unit and maintain its patency. The patency may be affected by superimposed mucosal edema, closing the narrow infundibulum. The reason why the infundibulum is narrow remains to be answered. Does the proximity of the infundibular walls create a distance between the mucosa which allows for the most efficient efflux of secretions from the sinuses in the normal individual?

Concha bullosa

Concha bullosa was found in the middle turbinate in 4/96, 4.2% of patients. Three had bilateral concha bullosa and one only on the left side. The size was not determined.

These results indicate the prevalence of concha

bullosa to be quite low in the pediatric population. Concha bullosa has been reported to be anatomically associated with an increased incidence of sinus disease. Since we studied children who had no or minimal sinus disease, we can only conclude that the prevalence of this anatomical variant is less than is seen in adults.

CONCLUSIONS

The results of our study have implications for the endoscopic and for the microscopic sinus surgeon. Knowledge of the developmental anatomy of the ostiomeatal unit and surrounding structures is important for safe functional sinus surgery in children. In our study, we have attempted to quantitate this development by examining several parameters.

In conclusion, we feel that the ostiomeatal unit is readily identifiable radiographically in children through the use of computerized tomographic imaging. There appears to be predictable linear growth of the ethmoid sinus system and upper nasal cavity width. Little change occurs within the ostiomeatal unit itself in terms of the infundibular width and uncinate angle. There appears to be an early growth pattern of the nasal cavity in terms of height, with a plateau in the later childhood years. And, finally, there appears to be an increased prevalence of Haller's cells and a decreased prevalence of concha bullosa in the pediatric population.

We hope that our results provide further insight into the understanding of the development of the ostiomeatal complex in childhood, and that some of the measurements may be useful to the functional sinus surgeon. We still feel, nevertheless, that preoperative assessment of coronal CT scans is of utmost importance in order to assess abnormal anatomy in each individual case. Identification of landmarks still remains the most important form of intraoperative guidance available to the functional sinus surgeon.

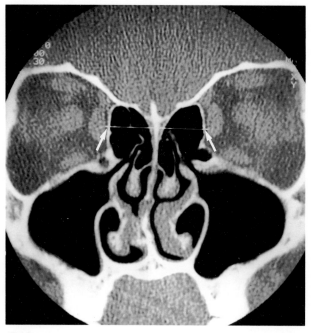

15.1A

AGE (years)	MEAN LAMINA–LAMINA distance (cm)
1–2	1.70
2–3	1.75
3–4	1.85
4–5	1.93
5–6	1.94
6–7	1.96
7–8	2.03
8–9	2.04
9–10	2.21
10–11	2.26
11–12	2.25
12–13	2.32
13–14	2.44
14–15	2.41
15–16	2.43

15.1B

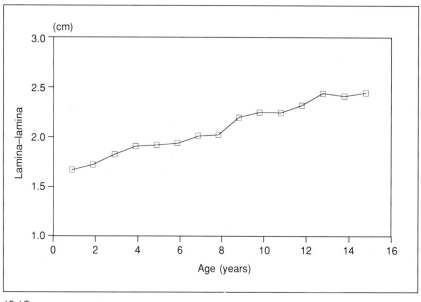

15.1C

Figure **15.1**

Interlaminar distance. (A) 3 mm coronal CT section of the ostiomeatal unit demonstrates the method for measuring the interlaminar distance (between arrows). (B) Mean for each age group. (C) The plotted data: note the linear rate of change.

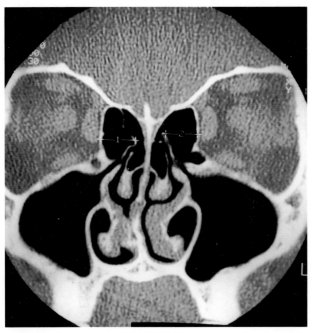

15.2A

AGE (years)	MEAN ANTERIOR ETHMOID WIDTH (cm)
1–2	0.39
2–3	0.40
3–4	0.50
4–5	0.55
5–6	0.48
6–7	0.53
7–8	0.65
8–9	0.63
9–10	0.62
10–11	0.60
11–12	0.69
12–13	0.75
13–14	0.79
14–15	0.76
15–16	0.78

15.2B

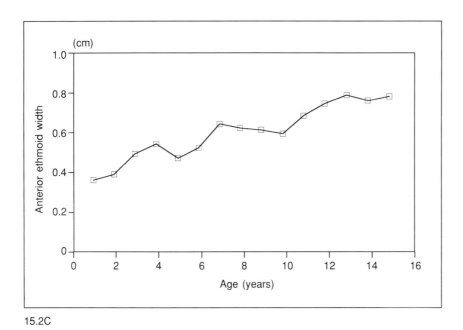

15.2C

Figure **15.2**

Anterior ethmoid width. (A) 3 mm coronal CT section of the ostiomeatal unit demonstrates the method for measuring the anterior ethmoid width. The lines shown are computer-generated graphics. (B) Mean for each age group. (C) The plotted data.

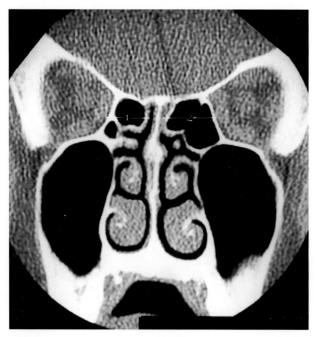

15.3A

AGE (years)	MEAN POSTERIOR WIDTH (cm)
1–2	0.48
2–3	0.56
3–4	0.67
4–5	0.72
5–6	0.78
6–7	0.78
7–8	0.90
8–9	0.89
9–10	0.89
10–11	0.93
11–12	0.87
12–13	0.96
13–14	1.04
14–15	1.09
15–16	1.10

15.3B

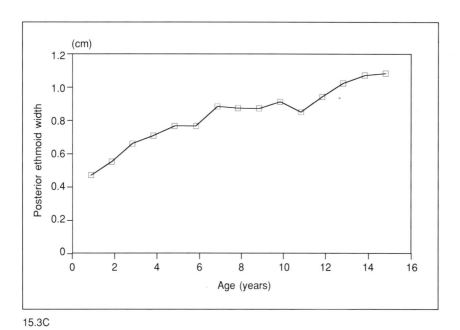

15.3C

Figure **15.3**

Posterior ethmoid width. (A) 3 mm coronal CT section of the ostiomeatal unit demonstrates the method for measuring the posterior ethmoid width. (B) Means for each age group. (C) The plotted data: note the linear rate of change.

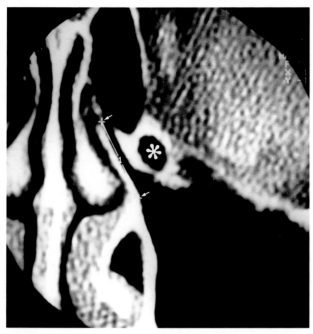

15.4A

AGE (years)	MEAN INFUNDIBULAR LENGTH (cm)
1–2	0.86
2–3	0.86
3–4	0.88
4–5	0.90
5–6	0.95
6–7	0.89
7–8	1.14
8–9	0.94
9–10	1.15
10–11	1.20
11–12	1.10
12–13	1.36
13–14	1.36
14–15	1.10
15–16	1.28

15.4B

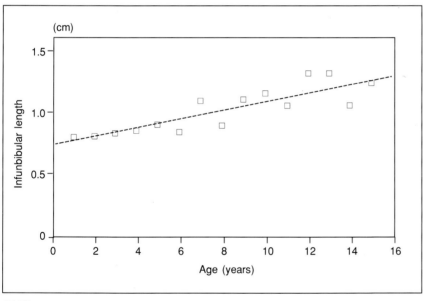

15.4C

Figure **15.4**

Infundibular length. (A) Magnified 3 mm CT section of the ostiomeatal unit demonstrates the method for measuring the infundibular length (between arrows). Note presence of Haller cell (asterisk). (B) Means for each age group. (C) The plotted data: note the variability.

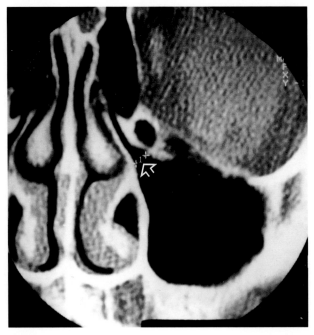

15.5A

AGE (years)	MEAN INFUNDIBULAR WIDTH (cm)
1–2	0.19
2–3	0.18
3–4	0.19
4–5	0.20
5–6	0.19
6–7	0.20
7–8	0.18
8–9	0.19
9–10	0.19
10–11	0.22
11–12	0.22
12–13	0.21
13–14	0.20
14–15	0.21
15–16	0.22

15.5B

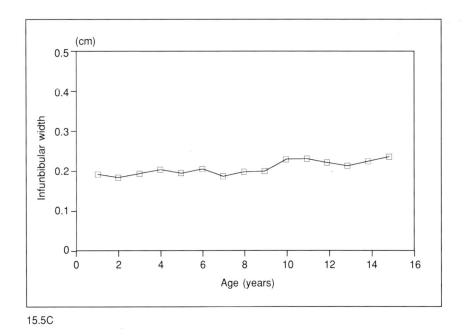

15.5C

Figure **15.5**

Infundibular width. (A) Magnified 3 mm CT section of the ostiomeatal unit demonstrates the method for measuring the infundibular width (open arrow). (B) Means for each age group. (C) The plotted data show little change in this parameter.

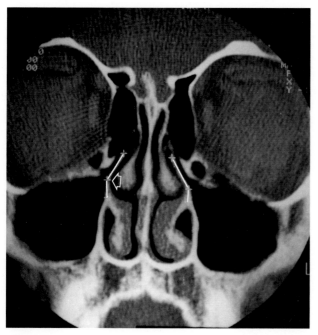

15.6A

AGE (years)	MEAN UNCINATE ANGLE (degrees)
1–2	146
2–3	149
3–4	145
4–5	142
5–6	145
6–7	145
7–8	148
8–9	143
9–10	140
10–11	146
11–12	140
12–13	140
13–14	141
14–15	139
15–16	141

15.6B

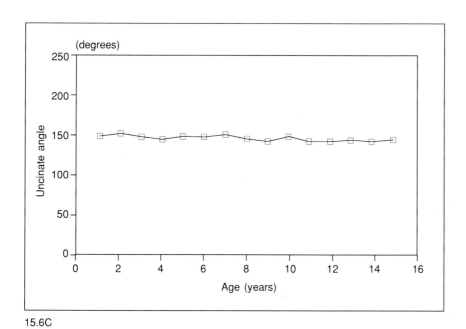

15.6C

Figure **15.6**

Uncinate angle. (A) 3 mm coronal CT section of the ostiomeatal unit demonstrates the method for measuring the uncinate angle. The angle indicated by the arrow was measured. (B) Means for each age group. (C) The plotted data: note the slight decrease.

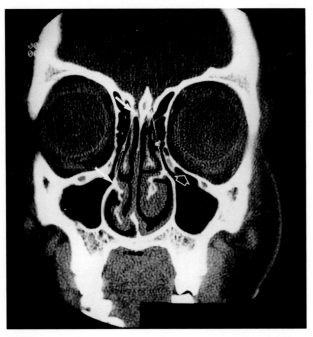

15.7A

AGE (years)	MEAN INFERIOR TURBINATE TO CRIBIFORM PLATE distance (cm)
1–2	1.76
2–3	1.93
3–4	1.91
4–5	2.07
5–6	2.11
6–7	2.34
7–8	2.28
8–9	2.32
9–10	2.47
10–11	2.49
11–12	2.48
12–13	2.58
13–14	2.53
14–15	2.51
15–16	2.56

15.7B

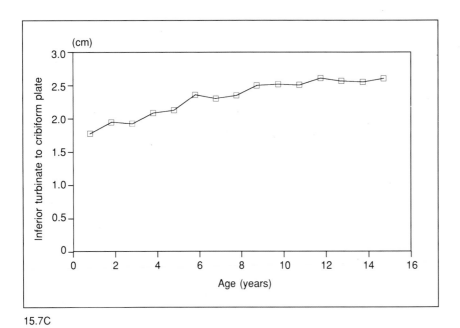

15.7C

Figure **15.7**

Distance between the inferior turbinate and cribriform plate. (A) 3 mm coronal CT section of the ostiomeatal unit demonstrates the method for measuring the distance from the inferior turbinate to the cribiform plate (between arrows). Note the pneumatized cell along the lateral wall of the infundibulum (open arrow). (B) Means for each age group. (C) The plotted data.

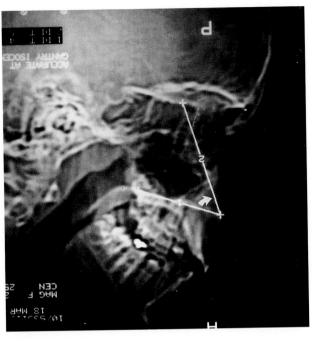

15.8A

AGE (years)	MEAN NASAL SPINE – ETHMOID FOVEOLA distance (cm)
1–2	3.38
2–3	3.60
3–4	4.05
4–5	4.40
5–6	4.48
6–7	4.48
7–8	4.61
8–9	4.73
9–10	4.90
10–11	5.12
11–12	5.34
12–13	5.45
13–14	5.52
14–15	5.50
15–16	5.51

15.8B

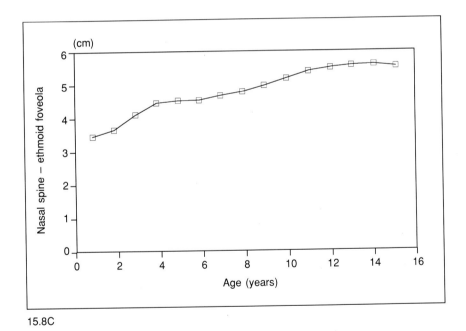

15.8C

Figure **15.8**

Distance between the anterior nasal spine and ethmoid roof.
(A) Scout film of the skull showing method of measuring the
distance between the nasal spine and the roof of the ethmoid
sinus. The angle indicated (curved arrow) is 55°. (B) Means for
each age group. (C) The plotted data: note the slope of the
curve.

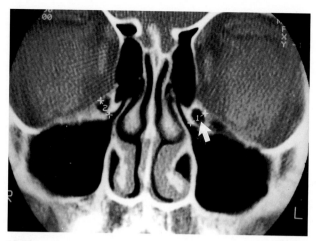

15.9A

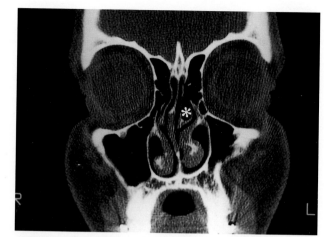

15.9B

Figure 15.9

Anatomic variants. (A) Coronal scan through the ostiomeatal
unit. Haller's cell present bilaterally (arrow). (B) This coronal
scan reveals the presence of a left middle turbinate concha
bullosa (asterisk).

Bibliography

Adams L, Krybus W, Meyer-Ebrecht D et al (1990) Computer assisted surgery, *IEEE Comput Graphics Appl* **10**(3):43–51.

Astor FC, Donegan O, Glugman JL (1985) Unusual anatomic presentations of inverting papilloma, *Head Neck Surg* **7**:243–5.

Balter S (1987) An introduction to the physics of magnetic resonance imaging, *Radiographics* **7**:371–83.

Babbel R, Harnsberger HR, Nelson B et al (1991) Optimization of techniques in screening CT of the sinuses, *AJNR* **12**:849–54.

Bassoiouny A, Newlands WJ, Ali H et al (1982) Maxillary sinus hypoplasia and superior orbital fissure asymmetry, *Laryngoscope* **92**:441–8.

Beahm E, Teresi L, Lufkin R et al (1990) MR of the paranasal sinuses, *Surg Radiol Anat* **12**:203–8.

Berlinger NT (1985) Sinusitis in immunodeficient and immunosuppressed patients, *Laryngoscope* **95**:29.

Bingham B, Shankar L, Hawke M (1991) Pitfalls in computed tomography of the paranasal sinuses, *J Otolaryngol* **20**(6):414–18.

Bolger WE, Woodruff WW, Morehead J (1990) Maxillary sinus hypoplasia: classification and description of associated uncinate process hypoplasia, *Otolaryngol Head Neck Surg* **103**:759–65.

Bolger WE, Butzin CA, Parsons DS (1991) Paranasal sinus bony anatomic variations and mucosal abnormalities: CT analysis for endoscopic sinus surgery, *Laryngoscope* **101**:56–64.

Bradley WG Jr (1984) Fundamentals of magnetic resonance image interpretation. In: Bradley WG, Adey WR, Hasso AN, eds, *Magnetic resonance imaging of the brain, head, and neck: a text atlas* (Rockville: Aspen) 1–16.

Bridger MWM, van Nostrand AWP (1978) The nose and paranasal sinuses — applied surgical anatomy, *J Otolaryngol* **7** (suppl 6).

Brockbank MJ, Brookes GB (1991) The sphenoiditis spectrum, *Clin Otolaryngol* **16**:15–20.

Buchwald C, Nielson LH, Ahlgren P et al (1990) Radiologic aspects of inverted papilloma, *Eur J Radiol* **10**:134–9.

Calhoun KH, Rotzler WH, Stiernberg CM (1990) Surgical anatomy of the lateral nasal wall, *Otolarnygol Head Neck Surg* **102**:156–60.

Carter BL, Bankoff MS, Fisk JD (1983) Computed tomographic detection of sinusitis responsible for intracranial and extracranial infections, *Radiology* **147**:739–42.

Catalano PJ, Lawson W, Som P et al (1990) Radiographic evaluation and diagnosis of the failed frontal osteoplastic flap with fat obliteration, *Otolaryngol Head Neck Surg* **104**:225–34.

Centeno RS, Bentson JR, Mancuso AA (1981) CT scanning in rhinocerebral mucormycosis and aspergillosis, *Radiology* **140**:383–9.

Conner BL, Roach ES, Laster W et al (1989) Magnetic resonance imaging of the paranasal sinuses: frequency and type of abnormalities, *Ann Allergy* **62**:457–60.

Cooke LD, Hadley DM (1991) MRI of the paranasal sinuses: incidental abnormalities and their relationship to symptoms, *J Laryngol Otol* **105**:278–81.

Crain MR, Dolan KD, Maves MD (1990) Maxillary sinus mucocele, *Ann Otol Rhinol Laryngol* **99**:321–2.

Curtin HD, Williams R (1985) Computed tomographic anatomy of the pterygopalatine fossa, *Radiographics* **5**(3):429–35.

Curtin HD, Williams R, Johnson J (1985) CT of perineural tumor extension: pterygopalatine fossa, *AJR* **144**:163–9.

Daniels DL, Rauschning W, Lovas J et al (1983) Pterygopalatine fossa: computed tomographic studies, *Radiology* **149**:511–16.

Daniels DL, Pech P, Kay MC et al (1985) Orbital apex: correlative anatomic and CT study, *AJR* **145**:1141–4.

Dillon WP, Som PM, Fullerton GD (1990) Hypointense MR signal in chronically inspissated sinonasal secretions, *Radiology* **174**:73–8.

Dodd GD, Jing BS (1977) *Radiology of the nose, paranasal sinuses and nasopharynx* (Williams and Wilkins: Baltimore).

Dolan KD, Smoker WRK (1983a) Paranasal sinus radiology, part 4A: maxillary sinuses, *Head Neck Surg* **5**:345–62.

Dolan K, Smoker WRK (1983) Paranasal sinus radiology, part 4B: maxillary sinus, *Head Neck Surg* **5**:428–46.

Drake JM, Joy M, Goldenberg A et al (1991) Computer- and robot-assisted resection of thalamic astrocytomas in children, *Neurosurgery* **29**(1):27–33.

Fascenelli FW (1969) Maxillary sinus abnormalities, *Arch Otolaryngol* **90**:98–101.

Friets EM, Strohbein JW, Hatch JF et al (1989) A frameless stereotactic operation microscope for neurosurgery, *IEEE Trans Biomed Eng* **36**:608–17.

Freedmann HM, Kern EB (1979) Complications of intranasal ethmoidectomy: a review of 1000 consecutive operations, *Laryngoscope* **89**:421–34.

Fullerton GD (1987) Magnetic resonance imaging signal concepts, *Radiographics* **7**:579–96.

Furin MJ, Zinreich SJ, Kennedy DW (1991) The atelectatic maxillary sinus, *Am J Rhinol* **5(3)**:79–83.

Gonsalves CG, Briant TDR (1978) Radiologic findings in nasopharyngeal angiofibromas, *J Can Assos Radiol* **29**:209–13.

Gray H (1973) *Gray's anatomy*, 35th edn, ed. Goss CM (Lea & Febiger: Philadelphia).

Grossman RJ, Gomori JM, Goldberg HL et al (1988) MR imaging of hemorrhagic conditions of the head and neck, *Radiographics* **8**:441–54.

Guthrie BL, Adler JR (1991) Frameless stereotaxy: computer assisted neurosurgery. In: Barrow, DL, ed, *Perspectives in neurological surgery*, vol 2 (Quality Medical Publications: St Louis).

Hasso AN (1984) CT of tumours and tumour like conditions of the paranasal sinuses, *Radiol Clin North Am* **22(1)**:119–30.

Havas TE, Motbey JÅ, Gullane PJ (1988) Prevalence of incidental abnormalities on computed tomographic scans of the paranasal sinuses, *Arch Otolaryngol Head Neck Surg* **114**:856–9.

Hunink MGM, de Slegte RGM, Gerritsen GJ et al (1990) CT and MR assessment of tumors of the nose and paranasal sinuses, the nasopharynx and the parapharyngeal space using ROC methodology, *Neuroadiology* **32**:220–5.

Jacobs M, Som PM (1982) The ethmoidal 'polypoidal mucocoele', *J Comput Assist Tomogr* **6(4)**:721–4.

Jorgensen RA (1991) Endoscopic and computer tomographic findings in ostiomeatal sinus disease, *Arch Otolaryngol Head Neck Surg* **117**:279–87.

Katsantonis GP, Friedman WH, Sivore MC (1990) The role of computed tomography in revision sinus surgery, *Laryngoscope* **100**:811–16.

Kelly PJ (1990) Stereotactic imaging, surgical planning and computer assisted resection of intracranial lesions: methods and results, *Adv Technical Stand Neurosurg* **17**:77–118.

Kennedy DW, Zinreich SJ, Rosenbaum AF et al (1985) Functional endoscopic sinus surgery: theory and diagnostic evaluation, *Arch Otolaryngol* **111**:576–82.

Kennedy DW, Zinreich SJ, Shaalan H et al (1987) Endoscopic middle meatal antrostomy: theory, technique and patency, *Laryngoscope* (suppl. 43, 97:8 III) 1–9.

Kennedy DW, Josephson JS, Zinreich SJ et al (1989) Endoscopic sinus surgery for mucocoeles: a viable alternative, *Laryngoscope* **99**:885–95.

Khanobthamchai K, Shankar L, Hawke M et al (1991a) The ethmomaxillary sinus and hypoplasia of the maxillary sinus, *J Otolaryngol* **20(6)**:425–7.

Khanobthamchai K, Shankar L, Hawke M et al (1991b) The secondary middle turbinate, *J Otolaryngol* **20(6)**:412–13.

Klimek L, Mösges R, Bartsch M (1991a) Indications for CAS (computer assisted surgery) systems as navigation aids in ENT-surgery. In: Lenke HU, Rhodes ML, Jaffe C et al, eds, *Proceedings of the CAR '91* (Springer-Verlag: Berlin) 358–61.

Klimek L, Wenzel M, Mösges R et al (1991b) Computergestütztes Verfahren zur intraoperativen Orientierung bei Orbitaeingriffen, *Ophtalmo-Chirurgie* **3**:177–83.

Kopp W, Stammberger H, Fotter R (1988) Special radiologic imaging of paranasal sinuses, *Eur J Radiol* **8**:153–6.

Kosugi Y, Watanabe E, Goto J (1988) An articulated neurosurgical navigation system using MRI and CT images, *IEEE Trans Biomed Eng* **35(2)**:147–52.

Kwoh YS, Hou J, Jonckheere EA et al (1988) A robot with improved absolute positioning accuracy for CT guided stereotactic brain surgery, *IEEE Trans Biomed Eng* **35(2)**:153–160.

Laborde G, Gilsbach J, Harders A et al (1992) CAL — a computer assisted localizer for preoperative planning of surgery and intraoperative orientation, *Acta Neurochir* in press.

Lang J (1990) *The clinical anatomy of the nasal cavity and paranasal sinuses* (Theime: Stuttgart).

Lauffer RB (1990) Magnetic resonance contrast media: principles and progress, *Magn Reson Q* **6**:65–84.

Lanzieri CF, Shah M, Krauss D et al (1991) Use of gadolinium-enhanced MR imaging for differentiating mucoceles from neoplasms in the paranasal sinuses, *Radiology* **178**:425–8.

Leggett WB, Greenberg MM, Gannon WE et al (1991) The viewing wand: a new system for three-dimensional computed tomography-correlated intraoperative localization, *Curr Surg* **48(10)**:674–8.

Lidov M, Behin F, Som PM (1990) Calcified sphenoid mucocoele, *Arch Otolaryngol Head Neck Surg* **116**:718–20.

Littlejohn MC, Stiernberg CM, Hokanson JA et al (1982) The relationship between the nasal cycle and mucociliary clearance, *Laryngoscope* **102**:117–20.

Lloyd GAS (1990) CT of the paranasal sinuses: study of a control series in relation to endoscopic sinus surgery, *J Laryngol Otol* **104**:477–81.

Lloyd GAS, Lund VJ, Phelps PD et al (1987) Magnetic resonance imaging in the evaluation of nose and paranasal sinus disease, *Br J Radiol* **60**:957–68.

Lund VJ, Lloyd GAS (1984) Radiological changes associated with inverted papilloma of the nose and paranasal sinuses, *Br J Radiol* **57**:455–61.

Mackay IS, Bull TR, eds (1987) *Scott Brown's otolaryngology, vol 4: rhinology*, 5th edn (London: Butterworths).

Mafee MF (1991) Endoscopic sinus surgery: role of the radiologist, *AJNR* **12**:855–60.

Maniglia AJ (1989) Fatal and major complications secondary to nasal and sinus surgery, *Laryngoscope* **99**:276–83.

Maran AGD, Lund VJ (1990) *Clinical rhinology* (Thieme: New York).

Masala W, Perugini S, Salvolini U et al (1989) Multiplanar reconstruction in the study of ethmoid anatomy, *Neuroradiology* **31**:151–5.

Messerklinger W (1978) *Endoscopy of the nose* (Urban and Schwarzenberg: Baltimore).

Mitchell MR, Tarr RW, Conturo CL et al (1986) Spin echo technique selection: basic principles for choosing MRI pulse sequence timing intervals, *Radiographics* **6**:245–60.

Modic MT, Weinstein WA, Berlin J et al (1980) Maxillary sinus hypoplasia visualised with computed tomography, *Radiology* **135**:383–5.

Moloney JA, Badham NJ, McRae A (1987) The acute orbit: preseptal (periorbital) cellulitis subperiosteal abscess and orbital cellulitis due to sinusitis, *J Laryngol Otol* **12**(suppl) 1–18.

Moser FG, Panush D, Rubin JS et al (1991) Incidental paranasal sinus abnormalities on MRI of the brain, *Clin Radiol* **43**:252–4.

Mösges R, Schlöndorff G (1988) A new imaging method for intraoperative therapy control in skull base surgery, *Neurosurg Rev* **11**:245–7.

Mösges R, Schlöndorff G, Klimek L et al (1989) CAS — computer assisted surgery. An innovative surgical technique in clinical routine. In: Lemke HU, ed, *CAR '89* (Springer-Verlag: Berlin) 413–15.

Moss AJ, Parson VL (1986) *Current estimates from the national health interview survey, United States — 1985* (Hyatsville, Maryland: National Centre for Health Statistics) 66–7.

Nass RL, Holliday RA, Reede DL (1989) Diagnosis of surgical sinusitis using nasal endoscopy and computed tomography, *Laryngoscope* **99**:1158–60.

Noyek A (1991) *Head and neck radiology* (JB Lippincott: Philadelphia).

Noyek AM, Zizmor J (1976) Radiology of the maxillary sinus after Caldwell–Luc surgery, *Otolaryngol Clin North Am* **9**:135–51.

Price JC, Zinreich SJ (1989) Computer-fabricated custom mandibular replacement prosthesis, *Laryngoscope* **99**(2):222–4.

Pace Balzan A, Shankar L (1991) Hawke M, Computed tomographic findings in atrophic rhinitis, *J Otolaryngol* **20**(6):428–32.

Rak KM, Newell JD, Yakes WJ et al (1990) Paranasal sinuses on MR images of the brain: significance of mucosal thickening, *AJNR* **11**:1211–14.

Raymond HW, Zwiebel WJ, Harnesberger HR, eds (1991) Essentials of screening sinus computed tomography, *Seminars in Ultrasound, CT, and MR* **12**(6):526–612.

Rauchfuss A (1990) Komplikationen der endonasalen Chirurgie der Nasennebenhöhlen — Spezielle Anatomie, Pathomechanismen, operative Versorgung, *HNO* **38**:309–16.

Reinhard H, Meyer H, Amrein E (1988) A computer-assisted device for the intraoperative CT-correlated localization of brain tumors, *Eur Surg Res* **20**:51–8.

Rice DH (1989) Basic surgical techniques and variations of endoscopic sinus surgery, *Otolaryngol Clin North Am* **22**:713–26.

Ritter FN (1978) *The paranasal sinuses: anatomy and surgical technique* (CV Mosby: St Louis).

Roberts DW, Strohbein JW, Hatch JF et al (1986) A frameless stereotaxic integration of computerized tomographic imaging and the operating microscope, *J Neurosurg* **65**:545–9.

Robinson JD, Crawford SC, Teresi LM et al (1989) Extracranial lesions of the head and neck: preliminary experience with Gd-DTPA-enhanced MR imaging, *Radiology* **172**:165–70.

Rohen JW, Yokochi C (1983) *Color atlas of anatomy* (Schattauer-Verlag: Stuttgart).

Rontal M, Rontal E (1991) Studying whole-mounted sections of the paranasal sinuses to understand the complications of endoscopic sinus surgery, *Laryngoscope* **101**:361–66.

Runge VM, Clanton JA, Herzer WA et al (1984) Intravascular contrast agents suitable for magnetic resonance imaging, *Radiology* **153**:171–6.

Runge VM, Wood ML, Kaufman DM et al (1988) The straight and narrow path to good head and spine MRI, *Radiographics* **8**:507–31.

Russell EJ, Czervionke L, Huckman M et al (1985) CT of the inferomedial orbit and the lacrimal drainage apparatus: normal and pathologic anatomy, *AJR* **145**:1147–54.

Saini S, Modic MT, Hamm B et al (1991) Advances in contrast-enhanced MR imaging, *AJR* **156**:235–54.

Schaeffer JP (1920) *The nose, paranasal sinuses, nasolacrimal passageways, and the olfactory organ in man* (McGraw-Hill: New York).

Schaeffer JP (1936) The clinical anatomy and development of the paranasal sinuses, *Pa Med* **39**:395–404.

Schatz CJ, Becker TS (1984) Normal and CT anatomy of the paranasal sinuses, *Radiol Clin North Am* **22**:107–118.

Schlöndorff G, Meyer-Ebrecht D, Mösges R et al (1987) CAS — computer assisted surgery, *Arch Otorhinolaryngol* **2**:45–6.

Shankar L, Hawke M (1991) Principles and objectives of functional endoscopic sinus surgery and CT of the paranasal sinuses, *ENT J* **4**:1–4.

Silver AJ, Beredes S, Bello JA et al (1987) The opacified maxillary sinus: CT findings in chronic sinusitis and malignant tumors, *Radiology* **163**:205–10.

Som PM (1985) CT of the paranasal sinuses, *Neuroradiology* **27**:189–201.

Som PM, Bergeron RT (1991) *Head and neck imaging*, 2nd edn (Mosby-Year Book: St Louis).

Som PM, Lawson W, Biller HF et al (1986a) Ethmoid sinus disease: CT evaluation in 400 cases. Part one: non-surgical patients, *Radiology* **159**:591–7.

Som PM, Lawson W, Biller HF et al (1986b) Ethmoid sinus disease: CT evaluation in 400 cases. Part two: post-operative findings, *Radiology* **159**:599–604.

Som PM, Sacher M, Lawson W et al (1987) CT appearance distinguishing benign nasal polyps from malignancies, *J Comput Assist Tomogr* **11(1)**:129–33.

Som PM, Shapiro MD, Biller HF et al (1988) Sinonasal tumors and inflammatory tissues: differentiation with MR imaging, *Radiology* **167**:803–8.

Som PM, Dillon WP, Fullerton GD et al (1989a) Chronically obstructed sinonasal secretions: observations on T1 and T2 shortening, *Radiology* **172**:515–20.

Som PM, Dillon WP, Sze G et al (1989b) Benign and malignant sinonasal lesions with intracranial extension: differentiation with MR imaging, *Radiology* **172**:763–6.

Som PM, Dillon WP, Curtin HD et al (1990) Hypointense paranasal sinus foci: differential diagnosis with MR imaging and relation to CT findings, *Radiology* **176**:777–81.

Som PM, Lawson W, Lidov MW (1991) Simulated aggressive skull base erosion in response to benign sinonasal disease, *Radiology* **180**:755–9.

Stammberger H (1986) Endoscopic endonasal surgery — concepts in treatment of recurring rhinosinusitis. I Anatomic and pathophysiologic considerations, *Otolaryngol Head Neck Surg* **94**:143–6.

Stammberger H (1991) *Functional endoscopic sinus surgery: the Messerklinger technique* (BC Decker: Philadelphia).

Stankiewicz JA (1987) Complications of endoscopic nasal surgery: occurrence and treatment, *Amer J Rhinol* **1**:45–49.

Stankiewics JA (1989) Complications of endoscopic sinus surgery, *Otolaryngol Clin North Am* **22(4)**:749–59.

Stevens JK, Trogadis JT (1984) Computer assisted reconstruction from serial electron micrographs: a tool for the systematic study of neuronal form and function, *Adv Cell Neurobiol* **5**:341–69.

Stevens JK, Trogadis JT (1990) Volume Investigation Laboratory, *Res Focus Toronto Hosp* **14**:1–9.

Stevens JK, Davis TL, Friedman N et al (1980) A systemic approach to reconstructing microcircuitry by electron microscopy of serial sections, *Brain Res Rev* **2**:265–93.

Tassel PV, Lee Y, Jing B et al (1985) Mucoceles of the paranasal sinuses: MR imaging with CT correlation, *AJR* **153**:407–12.

Teatini G, Simonetti G, Salvolini U et al (1987) Computerized tomography of the ethmoid, *Ann Otol Rhinol Laryngol* **96**:239–50.

Terrier F, Weber W, Ruenfenacht D et al (1985a) Anatomy of the ethmoid: CT, endoscopic and macroscopic, *Am J Roentgenol* **144**:493–500.

Terrier F, Weber W, Ruenfenacht D et al (1985b) Anatomy of the ethmoid: CT, endoscopic, macroscopic, *AJNR* **6**:77–84.

Toriumi DM, Berktold RE (1989) Multiple frontoethmoid mucocoeles, *Ann Otol Rhinol Laryngol* **98**:831–3.

Torrigiani CA (1913) *Arch Ital di Anat e di Embr* **12**:153–253.

Towbin R, Han BK, Kaufman RA et al (1986) Postseptal

cellulitis: CT in diagnosis and management, *Radiology* **158**:735–7.

Unger JM, Shaffer K, Duncavage JA (1984) Computed tomography in nasal and paranasal sinus disease, *Laryngoscope* **94**:1319–24.

Valvasorri GE, Potter GD, Hanafee WN et al (1982) *Radiology of the ear, nose and throat* (W.B. Saunders: Philadelphia).

Valvassori GE, Buckingham RA, Carter BL et al (1988) *Head and neck imaging* (Thieme: Stuttgart).

Van Alyea OE (1951) *Nasal sinuses: an anatomic and clinical consideration*, 2nd edn (Williams & Wilkins: Baltimore).

Van Tassell P, Lee YY, Jing BS et al (1989) Mucocoeles of the paranasal sinuses: MR with CT correlation, *Am J Roentgenol* **153**:407–12.

Vogi T, Dresel S, Bilaniuk LT et al (1990) Tumors of the nasopharynx and adjacent areas: MR imaging with Gd-DTPA, *AJNR* **11**:187–94.

Wallace R, Salazar JE, Cowles S (1990) The relationship between frontal sinus drainage and ostiomeatal complex disease: a CT study in 217 patients, *AJNR* **11**:183–6.

Watanabe E, Watanabe T, Manaka S et al (1987) Three-dimensional digitizer (neuronavigator): new equipment for computed tomography guided stereotaxic surgery, *Surg Neurol* **27**:543–7.

Watanabe E, Mayanagi Y, Kosugi Y et al (1991) Open surgery assisted by the neuronavigator, a stereotactic, articulated, sensitive arm, *Neurosurgery* **28**/6:792–800.

Weber AL (1988) Tumors of the paranasal sinuses, *Otolaryngol Clin North Am* **21**:439–54.

Weber AL (1988) Inflammatory diseases of the paranasal sinuses and mucoceles, *Otolaryngol Clin North Am* **21**:421–38.

Weber AL, Mikulis DK (1987) Inflammatory disorders of the paraorbital sinuses and their complications, *Radiol Clin North Am* **25(3)**:615–30.

Wigand ME (1981) Transnasale, endoskopische Chirurgie der Nasennebenhöhlen bei chronischer Sinusitis. III. Die endonasale Siebbeinausräumung, *HNO* **29**:287–93.

Wigand ME (1990) *Endoscopic surgery of the paranasal sinuses and the anterior skull base* (Thieme: Stuttgart).

Wigand ME, Steiner W (1978) Endonasal sinus surgery with endoscopical control: from radical operation to rehabilitation of the mucosa, *Endoscopy* **10**:255–60.

Woodham JD, Doyle PW (1991) Surgical landmarks and resections for safe performance of conservative endoscopic sinus surgery, *J Otolaryngol* **20(6)**:451–4.

Yanagisawa E, Smith HW (1976) Radiology of the normal maxillary sinus and related structures, *Otolaryngol Clin North Am* **9**:55–81.

Young RF (1987) Application of robotics to stereotactic neurosurgery, *Neurol Res* **9**:123–8.

Yousem DM, Galetta SL, Gusnard DA et al (1989) MR findings in rhinocerebral mucormycosis, *J Comput Assist Tomogr* **13(5)**:878–82.

Yousem DM, Kennedy DW, Rosenberg S (1991) Ostiomeatal complex risk factors for sinusitis: CT evaluation, *J Otolaryngol* **20(6)**:419–24.

Zimmerman RA, Bilaniuk LT, Hackney DB et al (1987) Paranasal sinus hemorrhage: evaluation with MR imaging, *Radiology* **162**:499–503.

Zinreich SJ (1990a) Paranasal sinus imaging, *Otolaryngol Head Neck Surg* **103**:863–9.

Zinreich SJ (1990b) Paranasal sinus imaging, *Radiology* **103(5)**:863–9.

Zinreich SJ, Kennedy DW, Rosenbaum AE et al (1987) Paranasal sinuses: CT imaging requirements for endoscopic surgery, *Radiology* **163**:769–75.

Zinreich SJ, Mattox DE, Kennedy DW (1988a) Concha Bullosa: CT evaluation, *J Comput Assist Tomogr* **12(5)**:778–84.

Zinreich SJ, Kennedy DW, Malat J et al (1988b) Fungal sinusitis: diagnosis with CT and MR imaging, *Radiology* **169**:439–444.

Zinreich SJ, Kennedy DW, Kumar AJ et al (1988c) MR imaging of the normal nasal cycle: comparison with sinus pathology, *J Comput Assist Tomogr* **12(6)**:1014–19.

Zinreich SJ, Kennedy DW, Long DM et al (1990a) 3-D applications in neuroradiology, *Hospimedica* **8(1)**:29–32.

Zinreich SJ, Wang H, Abdo F et al (1990b) 3-D CT improves accuracy of spinal trauma studies, *Diagn Imag* **6**:102–7.

Zizmor J, Noyek AMN (1979) The radiological diagnosis of maxillary sinus disease, *Otolaryngol Clin North Am* **9**:93–115.

Zweifel HJ, Reinhardt HF, Horstmann GA et al (1990) CT/MRI-korrelierte Stereometrie mit Ultraschall für Hirnoperationen, *Ultraschall Med* **11**:72–5.

Index

Page numbers in *italic* refer to the illustrations.